Single Point Acupuncture
CLINICAL TREATMENT
单穴针炎临床治疗

Sumiko Knudsen

Ph.d.
Practitioner.DK

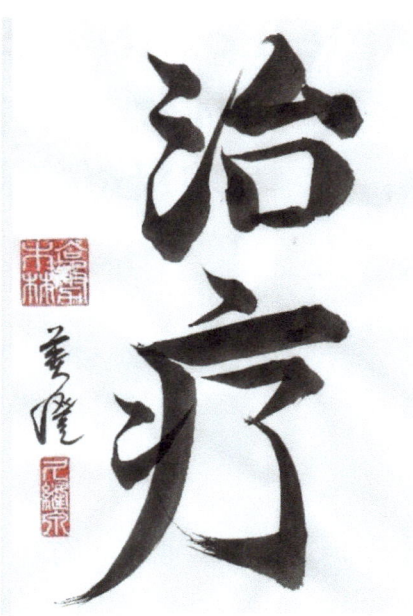

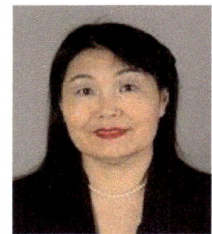

Sumiko Knudsen was born in Japan, and she has lived in USA, UK and Denmark for many years. She graduated at Nordic College of Chinese Acupuncture in Denmark, and then she went on and studied at Beijing University of TCM in China. After that she studied and graduated at Nanjing University of TCM in China. and she earned Ph.D. She is a private practitioner in Denmark.

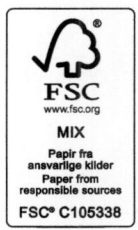

© 2024 Sumiko Knudsen
Forlag: BoD – Books on Demand, Hellerup, Danmark
Tryk: BoD – Books on Demand, Norderstedt, Tyskland

ISBN: 9788743058380

CONTENTS

INTRODUCTION

The Single point therapy is a significant therapy in Traditional Chinese Medicine. Using the Single point therapy has the characteristics of good curative effects.

In Therapeutics of acupuncture, acupuncture points are the places where acupuncture needle is applied for the treatment of diseases. The acupuncture point location and the therapeutic result are related.

The processing is done by inserting thin disposable needles into specific point relating to the internal organs. In this way body is activated with flow of Qi (energy).

This book guides by the principles governing the prescription and combination of points of Acupuncture, and it lets to find easily acupuncture points of diseases.

The locations of acupuncture points are certainly related to physiological functions. Stimulating acupoints in meridians of the affected area may be effective and stimulate meridian points for each disease to approach the affected area. Stimulation through acupuncture point can correct imbalance and blockages in the flow of energy for restoring health.

Sumiko Knudsen 克努森澄子

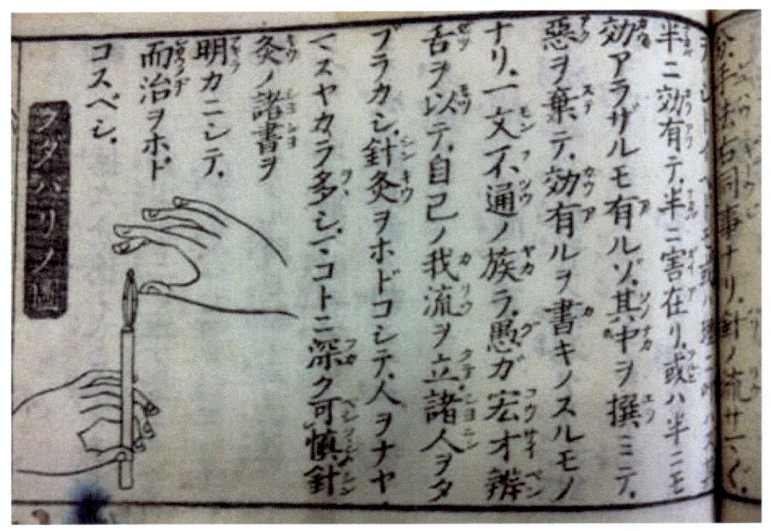

半ニ効有テ、半ニ害在リ、或ハ半ニヲ
効アラザルモ有ルゾ、其中ヲ撰ミテ、
悪ヲ棄テ、効有ルヲ書キノスルモノ
ナリ、一文ニ不通ノ族ヲ悪ガ宏才辨
舌ヲ以テ、自己ノ我流ヲ立諸人ヲ立タ
ブラカシ、針灸ヲホドコシテ、人ヲナヤ
マスヤカラ多シデ、コトニ深ク可懼針
灸ノ諸書ヲ
明カニシテ、
而治ヲホド
コスベシ。

フダバリノ圖

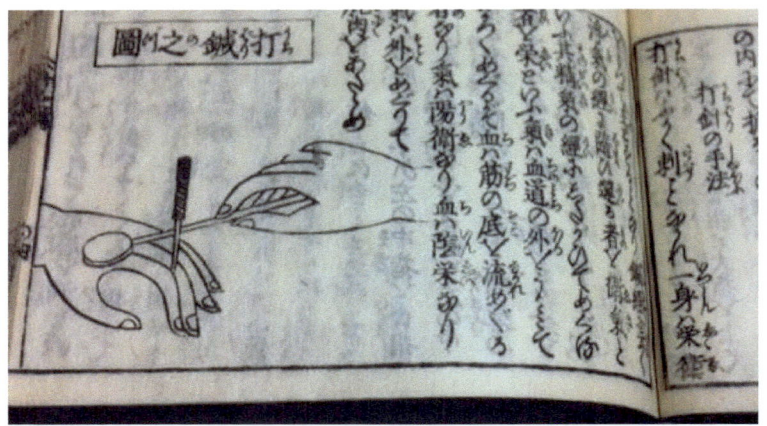

鍼打之圖

Edo period about 1600

Chapter 1 Internal Medicine
1-1 Abdominal pain 腹痛 Futong

It is caused by internal accumulation of cold. Sudden violent pain which responds to warmth and is aggravated by cold. Other manifestations include loose stools, profuse clear urine, white coated tongue, deep tense or deep slow pulse.

- **Treatment**
  Prescriptions

- **Main point**
  P-6 (内关 Neiguan)
- Luo-Connecting point of the Pericardium channel.
- On the palmar side of the forearm, 2 cun above the transverse crease of the wrist, on the line connecting P-3 (Quze 曲泽) and P-7 (Daling 大陵), between the tendons of palmaris longus and flexor carpi radialis.

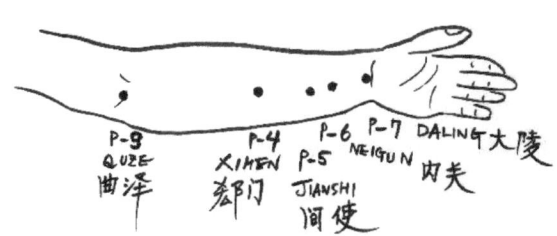

Secondary point
ST-36 (足三里 Zusanli)

- He-Sea point of the Stomach channel.
- 3 cun inferior to ST-35 (Dubi 犊鼻), one finger-breadth (middle finger) lateral to the anterior crest of the tibia.

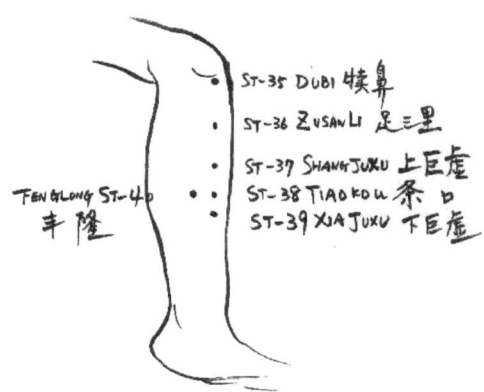

1-2 Stomach pain by food poisoning
Weitongshiwuzhongdu 胃痛食物中毒

It is food poisoning and stomach hurts badly.

- **Treatment**
  Prescriptions
- **Main point**
  EX (Lineiting 里内庭)

  This Ex point is directly **sole side/** of ST-44.

  *ST-44... On the dorsum of the foot, between the second and third toes, at the end of the vertical slin crease of the web.

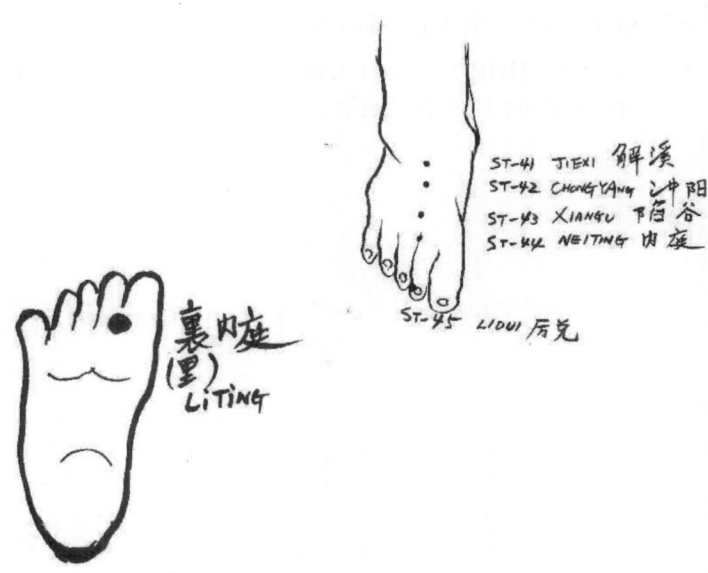

ST-41 JIEXI 解溪
ST-42 CHONGYANG 沖阳
ST-43 XIANGU 陷谷
ST-44 NEITING 内庭

ST-45 LIDUI 厉兑

裏内庭
(里)
LiTING

1-3 Stomach cramps 胃痉挛 Weijingluan

Stomach cramps are a condition in which the stomach contracts abnormally and is accompanied by severe pain. The cause is stress or an imbalance in the nervous system.

- **Treatment**
  Prescription

- **Main point**
  ST-34 (Liangqiu 梁丘**)**
- Xi-Cleft point of the Stomach channel.
- On the thigh, 2 cun above the superiolateral border of the patella.

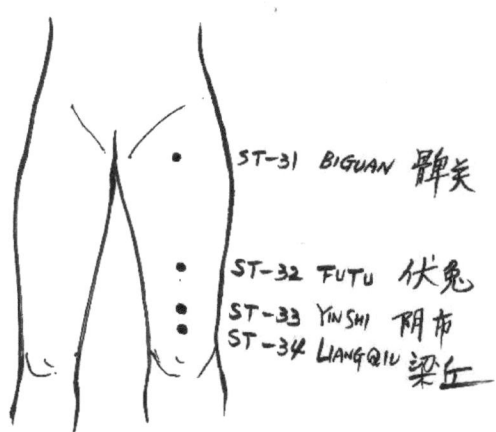

ST-31 BIGUAN 髀关

ST-32 FUTU 伏兎

ST-33 YIN SHI 阴市
ST-34 LIANGQIU 梁丘

1-4 Stomach heaviness 胃沉重 Weichenzong

A heavy stomach comes from indigestion.
It helps improve not only the function of the stomach, but also the digestive system, including the small intestine, diaphragm, and large intestine.

- **Treatment**
  Prescription

- **Main point**
  ST-45 (Lidui 厉兑)
- On the lateral side of the 2nd toe, 0.1 cun beside the corner of the nail.

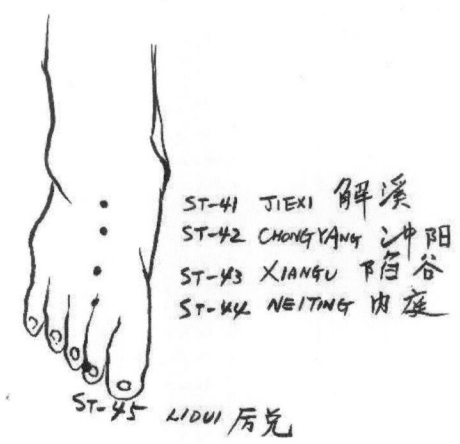

ST-41 JIEXI 解溪
ST-42 CHONGYANG 冲阳
ST-43 XIANGU 陷谷
ST-44 NEITING 内庭

ST-45 LIDUI 厉兑

1-5 Asthma 哮喘 Xiaochuan

This is attacked with different antigens, which is pollen, dust, shrimp fur.The pathogenical characteristics are muscle edema, bronchospasm, and bronchial obstruction. These are attacked with wheezing and expiratory dysnea.

- **Treatment**
  Prescription
- **Main point**
  REN-17 (Shanzhong 膻中)
- Front-Mu point of the Pericardium.
- At the level of the fourth intercostal space, the midpoint of the line connecting both nipples.

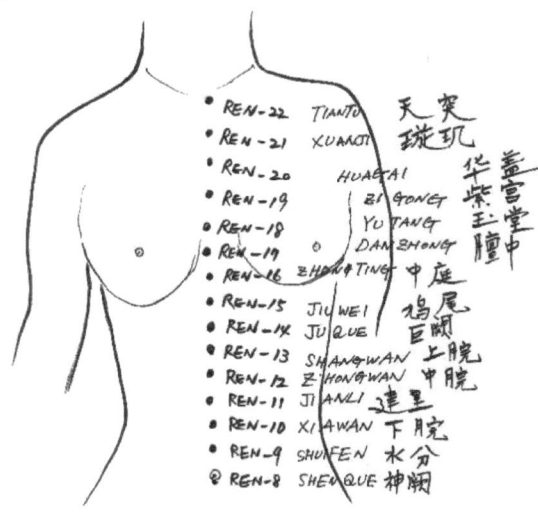

1-6 Bronchitis 支气管炎 Zhiqiguanyan

This is inflammation of the trachea or bronchi caused by bacterium, virus, physical, and chemical irritation. It usually has symptoms of fever, aversion to cold and infection of the upper respiratory tract. The main symptom is cough.

- **Treatment**
  Prescription

- **Main point**
  REN 22 (Tiantu 天突)
- On the neck, in the centre of the suprasternal fossa.

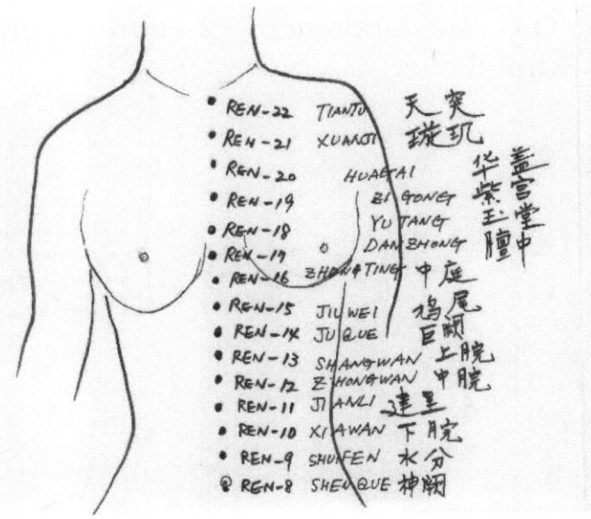

1-7 Constipation 便秘 Bianmi

Colon contractions become weak and abdominal muscle strength decreases, then leading to constipation. When this peristaltic movement becomes impaired, stool accumulates in the intestines, absorbs water, and becomes hard and difficult to pass.

- **Treatment**
  Prescription
- **Main point**
  ST-25 (Tianshu 天枢)
- Front-Mu point of the Large Intestine.
- On the abdomen, 2 cun lateral to the umbilicus.

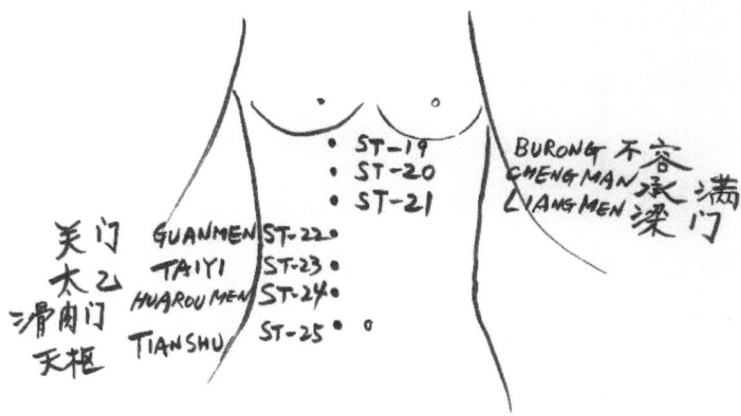

1. Secondary point
LI-2 (Erjian 二间)

- On the radial side of the index finger, in the depression distal to the second metacarpal-phalangeal joint. Point locates slightly flexed.

- Activates intestinal motility and restores normal intestinal function。

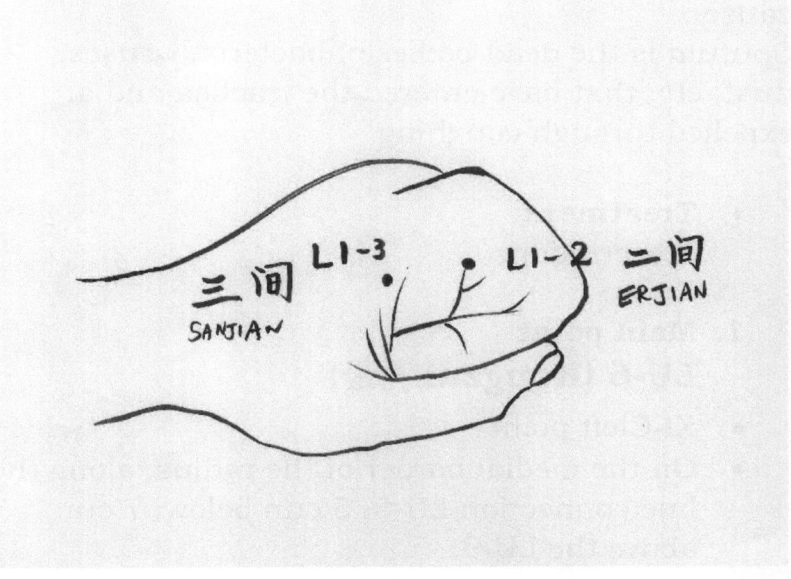

1-8 Cough and Phlegm 咳嗽有痰 Kesouyoutan

Coughing and sputum come from the back of the throat, larynx, trachea, and bronchi.

Coughing is an important function that reflexively expels foreign substances and exudates that have entered the throat and trachea. In addition, there are coughs that occur due to inflammation of the mucous membranes. It also happens from mental cause.

Sputum is the dead bodies of bacteria, viruses, dust, etc. that have entered the trachea and are expelled through coughing.

- **Treatment**
  Prescription

1. **Main point**
   LU-6 (Kongzui 孔最)

- Xi-Cleft point
- On the medial border of the radius, along the line connection LU-5, 5 cun below. 7 cun above the LU-9.

- LU-6 is transmitted to the central nervous system and helps to effectively eliminate phlegm.

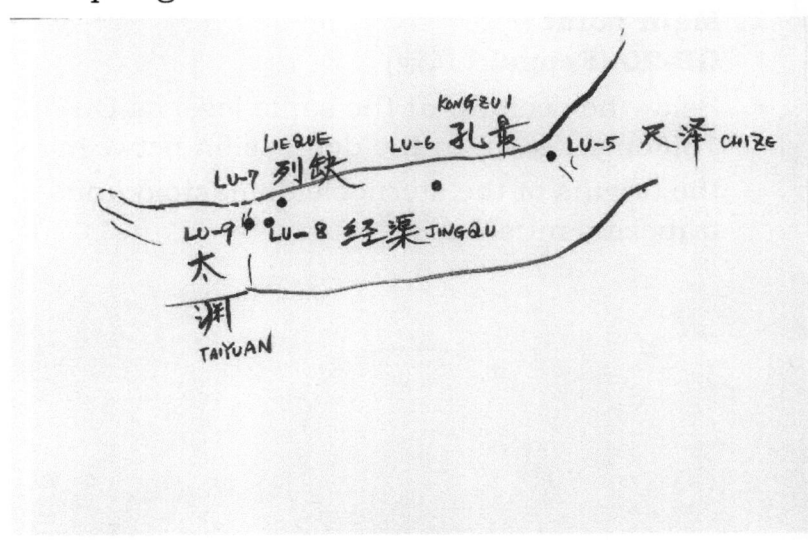

1-9 Common Cold 普通感 Putongganmao

Common cold has 3 types, Wind-cold type, Wind-heat type, and Damp-heat type. Clinically, it manifests as nasal obstruction, headache, running nose, cough, aversion to cold, sore throat, hoarse voice, etc. It accompanied with mild fever, lassitude etc.

- **Treatment**
  Prescription

1. Main point
GB-20 (Fengchi 凤池)

- Below he occiput, at the same level as Du-16(Fengfu 风府), in the depression between the origins of the sternocleidomastoid and trapezius muscles.

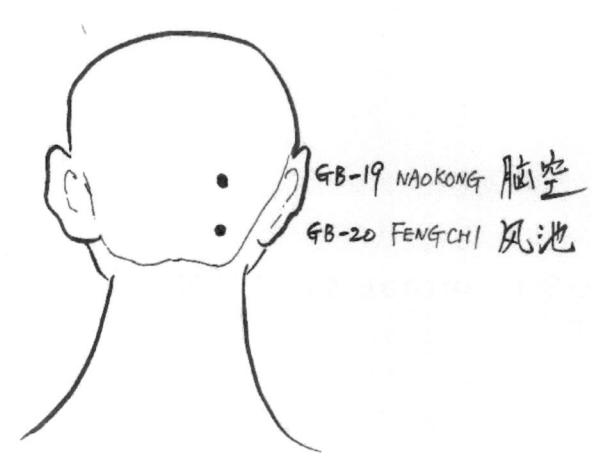

GB-19 NAOKONG 脑空

GB-20 FENGCHI 风池

2. Secondary point
DU-14 (Dazhui 大椎)

- Point of the Sea of Qi.

- Meeting point of the Governing vessel with Six Yang channel.
- At the level of the shoulder, in the depression below the spinous process of the seventh cervical vertebra.

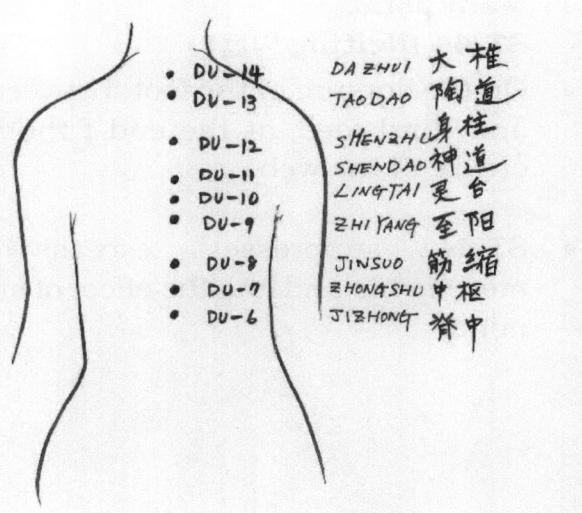

DU-14	DA ZHUI	大椎
DU-13	TAO DAO	陶道
DU-12	SHENZHU	身柱
DU-11	SHENDAO	神道
DU-10	LINGTAI	灵台
DU-9	ZHI YANG	至阳
DU-8	JINSUO	筋缩
DU-7	ZHONGSHU	中枢
DU-6	JIZHONG	脊中

1-10 Diarrhea 泄泻 Xiexie

Causes of diarrhea include food poisoning, colds, and stress.

The intestinal mucosa is stimulated for some reason, and the autonomic nerves abnormally increase intestinal motility. The time that stool remains in the large intestine is shortened, and the water is released without being absorbed.

- **Treatment**
  Prescription

1. Main point
ST-44 (Neiting 内庭)

- On the dorsum of the foot, between the second and third toes, at the end f the vertical skin crease of the web.

- ST-44 suppresses excessive intestinal movements and has the effect of stabilizing the mind.

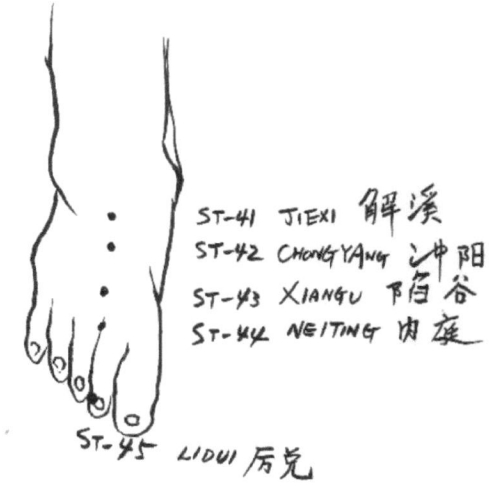

ST-41 JIEXI 解溪
ST-42 CHONGYANG 冲阳
ST-43 XIANGU 陷谷
ST-44 NEITING 内庭

ST-45 LIDUI 厉兑

1-11 Dizziness 眩暈 Xuanyun

The hearing organs and balance organs in the left and right inner ears are filled with lymph, which maintains balance and balance. When this breaks down, dizziness occurs.

Dizziness can also be caused by stiff shoulders, impaired blood flow in the blood vessels that supply nutrients to the inner ear, hormonal imbalance during menopause, overwork, or stress.

The key to treatment for dizziness is to identify the cause, improve it, and improve blood flow to the inner ear.

- **Treatment**
  Prescription

1. **Main point**
   P-6 (Neiguan 内关)
- Luo-Connecting point of the Pericardium channel.
- On the palmar side of the forearm, 2 cun above the transverse crease of the wrist, on the line connecting P-3 (Quze 曲泽) and P-7 (Daling 大陵), between the tendons of palmaris longus and flexor carpi radialis.

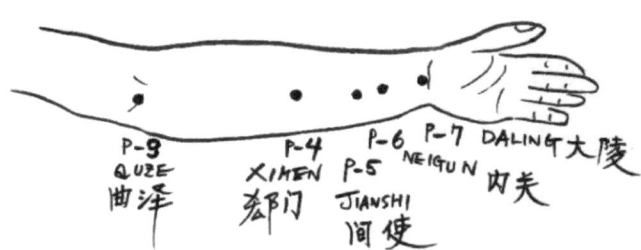

2. Secondary point
DU-20 (Baihui 白会)

- Point of the Sea of Marrow.
- On the midline of the head, 5 cun above the midpoint of the anterior hairline, at the midpoint connecting the apexes of both ears.

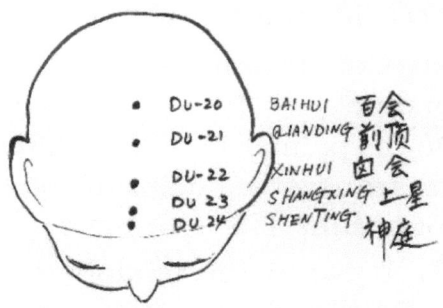

3. Moxibustion

1-12 Epilepsy 癫痫 Dianxian

This is defined as paroxysmal and temporary disturbance of brain characterized by loss of consciousness and muscle tic or abnormal sensation, emotion or behavior. It is characterized by sudden loss of consciousness, general spasm, foam in the mouth about 5 min. The patient may fall into sleep about few hours. This is accompanied with interruptions of speech and action, but usually comes to consciousness quickly.

- **Treatment**
  Prescription

- **Main point**
  DU-14 (Dazhui 大椎)
- Point of the Sea of Qi.
- Meeting point of the Governing vessel with Six Yang channel.
- (Regulating any Qi in the 6 Yang meridian, therefore regulating the brain.)

- At the level of the shoulder, in the depression below the spinous process of the seventh cervical vertebra.

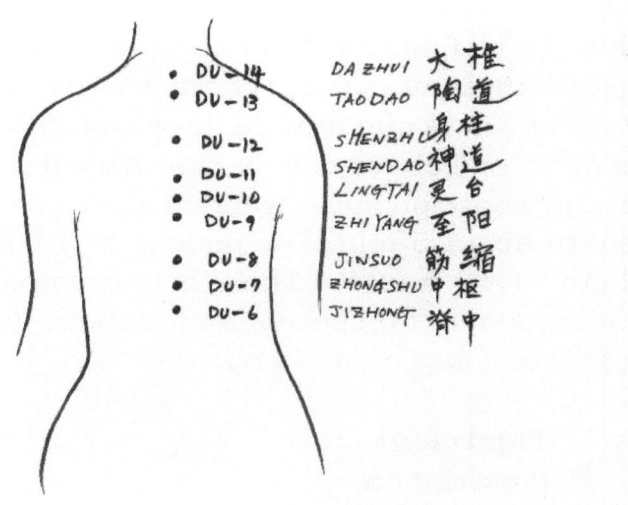

1-13 Gastritis 胃炎 Weiyan

It may be divided into the superficial, atrophic and hypertrophic according to its pathogenic changes. Clinical manifestations are epigastric pain, anorexia and indigestion.

- **Treatment**
  Prescription

- **Main point**

RN-12 (Zhongwan 中脘)

- Front-Mu point of the Stomach.
- On the upper abdomen, 4 cun above the umbilicus.

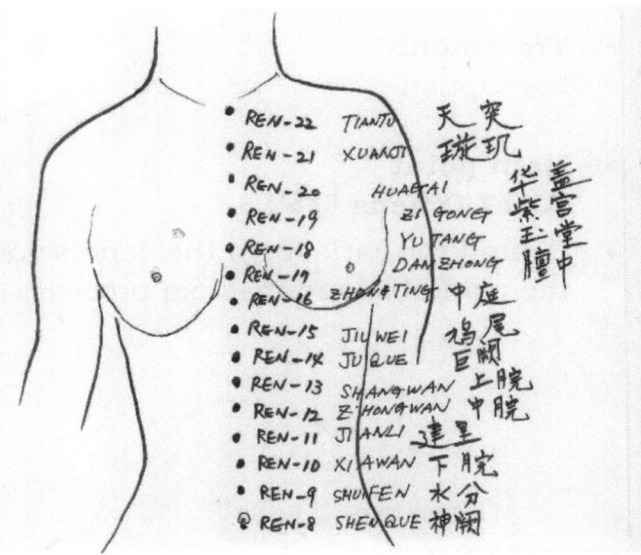

1-14 Hiccup 呃逆 Eni

Hiccup rises from:
- Retention of food and stagnation of Qi
  Epigastric and abdominal distension, sticky, yellow tongue coating, rolling forceful pulse.

- Attack by pathogenic Cold
  Alleviated by hot drinks, white moist tongue coating, slow pulse.

- **Treatment**
  Presription

- **Main point**
  SJ-17 (Yifeng 翳风)
- Behind the earlobe, in the depression between the mandible and mastoid process.

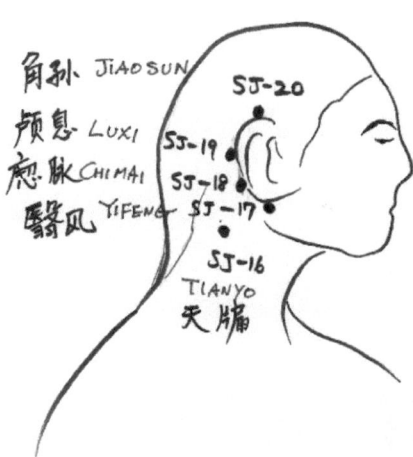

1-15 Hemorrhoids 痔疮 Zhichuang

There are two types of hemorrhoids:
wart hemorrhoids and fissure hemorrhoids. There are two sphincters in the anus: an outer and an inner sphincter.
When you strain to defecate, the tip of the intestine protrudes from the anus, and the sphincter muscle tightens on it, causing congestion and wart-like formations.
Hemorrhoids are those that tear and bleed when you defecate. Both are very painful.

Hemorrhoids occur when blood flow to the intestines and buttocks is poor.
If you sit for a long time or stay in a cold place, the blood flow around your intestines and buttocks becomes poor, and your muscles become weaker.

On the other hand, if the blood flow around the buttocks is good, the intestines will be elastic, warts will not form, and there will be no tears.

- **Treatment**
  Priscriptions
- **Main point**
  ST-37 (Shangjuxu 上巨虚)

- Lower He-Sea point of the Large Intestine.
- On the lower leg, 6 cun inferior to ST-35 (Dubi 犊鼻), one finger- breadth (middle finger) lateral to the anterior crest of the tibia.
- ST-37 improves blood circulation around the buttocks and relieves hemorrhoid pain.

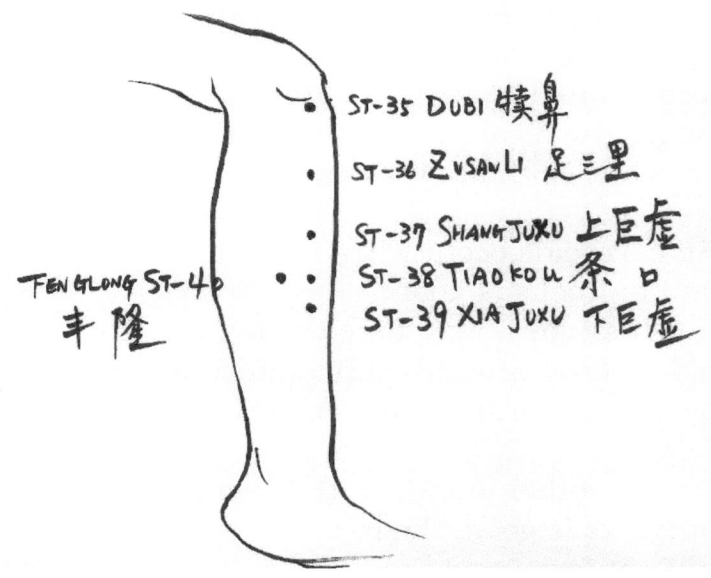

- **Secondary point**
  LU-6 (Kongzui 孔最)
- Xi-Cleft point

- On the medial border of the radius, along the line connection LU-5, 5 cun below. 7 cun above the LU-9.

- LU-6 has a hemostatic effect of acupuncture point that can be relieved well.

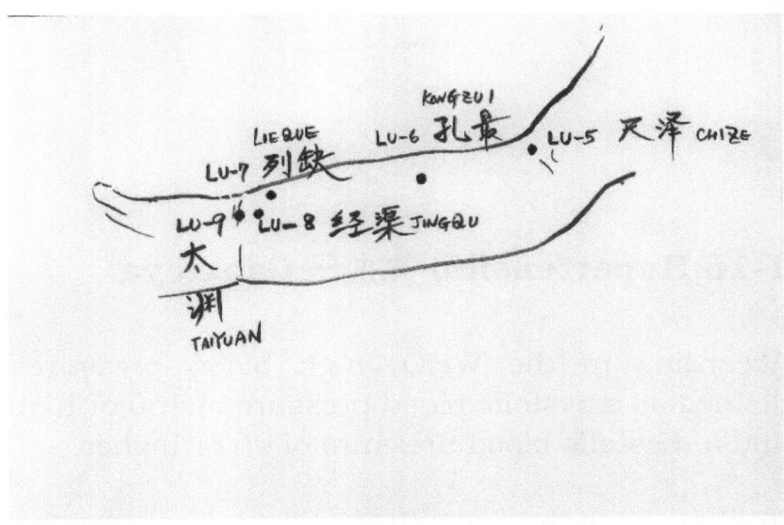

- **Third point**
  EX-UE2 (Erbai 二白)
- On the palmar side of forearm, a pair of points, 4 cun above the transverse crease of the wrist, on both sides of the tendon of m. flexor carpi radialis, two points on the hand.

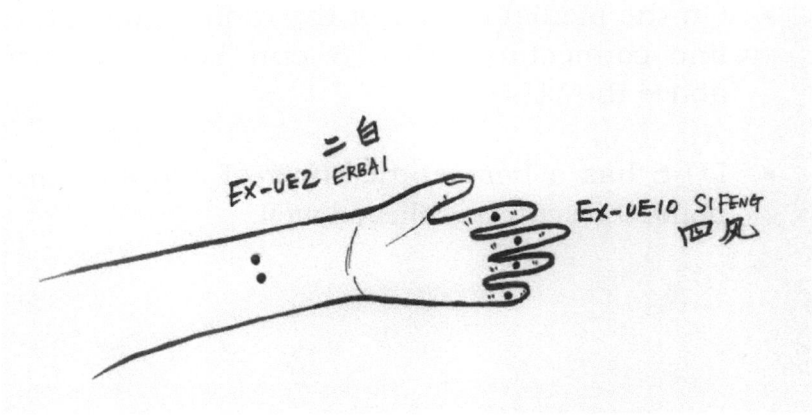

1-16 Hypertension 高血压 Gaoxieya

According to the WHO, high blood pressure is defined as a systolic blood pressure of 160 or higher and a diastolic blood pressure of 96 or higher.

In general, it is natural for blood pressure to be higher than normal when you are exercising or thinking. At such times, your body needs blood, so it is natural that blood flow increases and becomes higher. If your blood pressure is high or low when you are at rest, it means that your blood pressure is not normal.

In the early stage, there are symptoms of dizziness, headache, palpitation, insomnia, tinnitus, dysphoria, lassitude, etc. In the late stage, such as the heart, brain, kidneys, and others may be involved.

- **Treatment**
  Prescription

- **Main point**
  GB-39 (Xuanzhong 悬钟)
- On the lateral side of the lower leg, 3 cun superior to the prominence of the lateral malleolus, on the anterior border of the fibula.

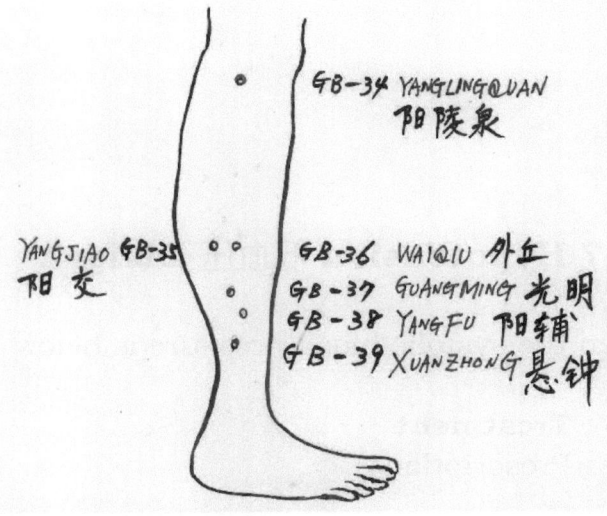

- **Secondary point**

REN-8 (Shenque 神阙)

In the centre of the umbilicus.

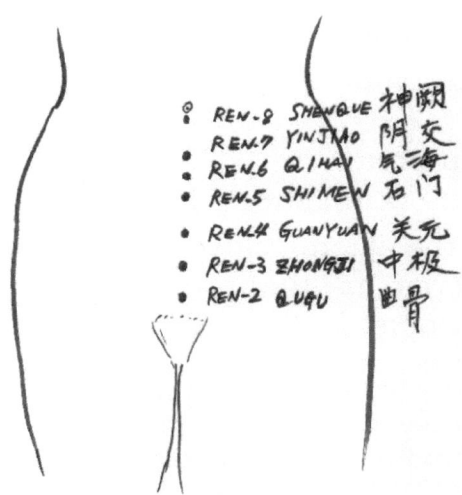

1-17 Hypotension 低血压 Dixieya

When the systolic blood pressure is below 100.

- **Treatment**
  Prescription

- **Main point**

GB-39 (Xuanzhong 悬钟)

- On the lateral side of the lower leg, 3 cun superior to the prominence of the lateral malleolus, on the anterior border of the fibula.

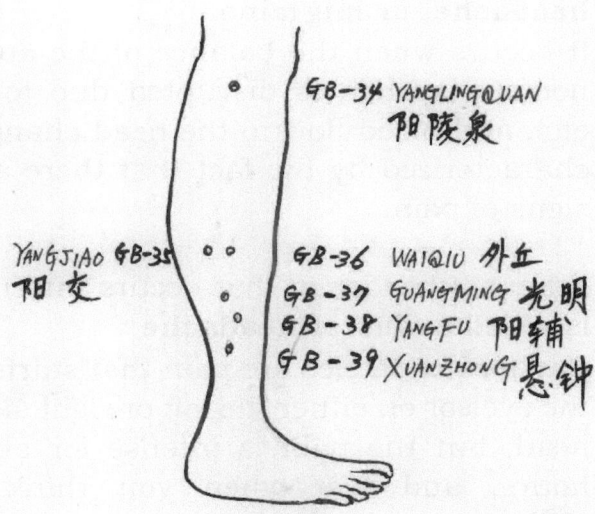

1-18 Headache 头痛 Toutong

1. Types of headaches

(1) Pain that feels like your head is being squeezed is called **a strangulation headache or a tension headache.**

- Stiffness in the neck and shoulders is caused by muscle tension. This is caused by lack of oxygen in the muscles and tired eyes.

(2) This is called **a throbbing pain, pulsating headache, or migraine.**
- It occurs when the balance of the autonomic nervous system is disrupted due to fatigue, etc., and blood flow to the head changes. It is characterized by the fact that there are often signs of pain.

(3) A type of headache that occurs intermittently is called **a cluster headache**.
- Cluster headaches are pain that starts behind the eyes or on either the left or right side of the head, but the pain is intense for about 1-2 hours, and just when you think it has subsided, the pain starts again. It happens repeatedly over several days, several times a day. The cause is overwork and stress; there is no abnormality in the brain, and it is not related to high blood pressure.

- **Treatment**
  Prescription

- **Main point**
  GB-36 (Waiqiu 外丘)
- Xi-Cleft point of the Gall Bladder channel.
- On the lateral aspect of the lower leg, 7 cun superior to the prominence of the lateral malleolus, on the anterior border of the fibula.

- GB-36 seems to stimulate the autonomic nervous system and balance blood flow. When blood flow improves, stiffness will also be removed. It can also prevent headaches.

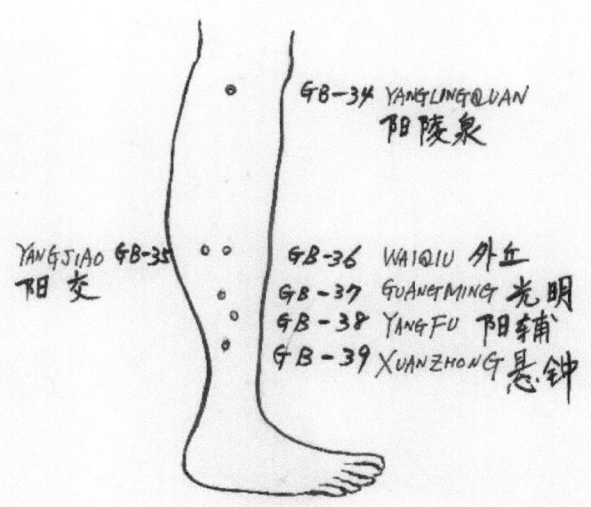

2. Headache region

(1) Occipital Headache
(2) Frontside Headache
(3) One-side Headache
(4) Parietal Headache

- **Secondary point
  (1) GB-20 (Fengchi 风池)**
- Below the occiput, at the same level as Du-16 (Fengfu 风府), in the depression between the origins of the sternocleidomastoid and trapezius muscles.

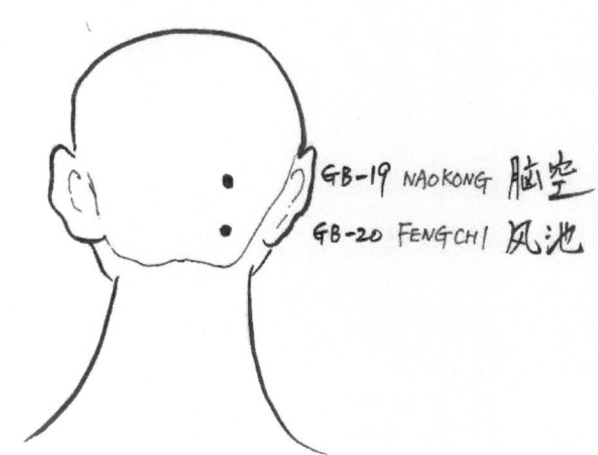

(2) BL-60 (Kunlun 昆仑)

- Behind the ankle joint, in the depression between the prominence of the lateral malleolus.

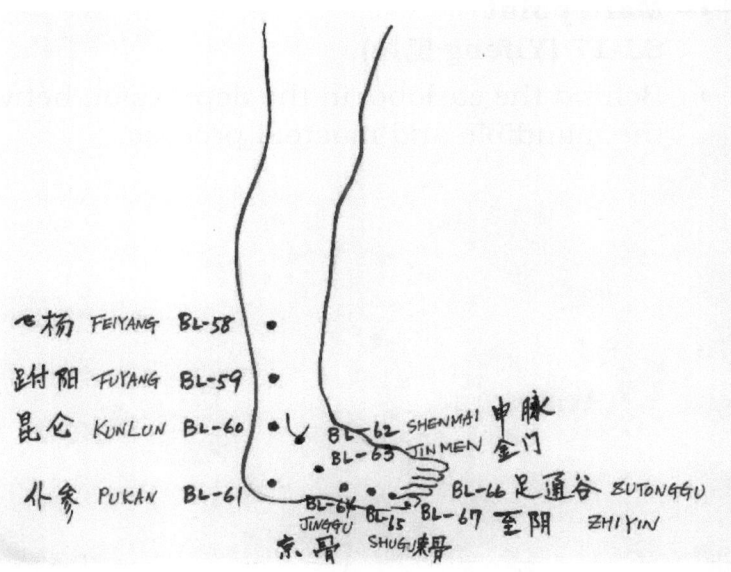

1-19 Migraine 偏头痛 Piantoutong

It causes sometimes, such as fatigue, poor sleep, and tension etc. There are attacks of burning on temple, on the forehead in most cases. The pain lasts for a few minutes and several days, and sometimes several times a day.

- **Treatment**
  Prescription

- **Main point**
  SJ-17 (Yifeng 翳风)
- Behind the earlobe, in the depression between the mandible and mastoid process.

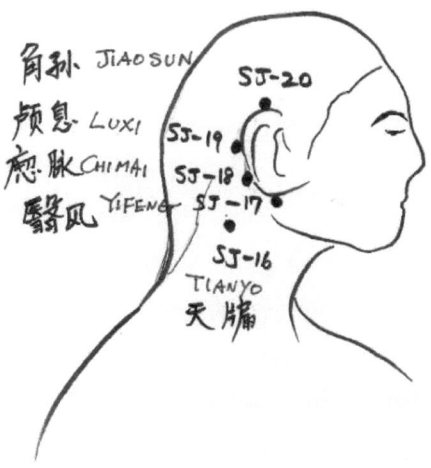

1-20 Insomnia 不寐 Bumei

3 types of sleeplessness

(1) It's difficult to fall asleep. A normal person can fall asleep in about 15 minutes but can't fall asleep for more than an hour.

(2) This is called waking up in the middle of the night, or difficulty falling asleep in the middle of the night.

(3) wake up early in the morning.

- **Treatment**
  Prescription

- **Main point**
  EX (Shimian 失眠)
- The point at the middle of the heel.

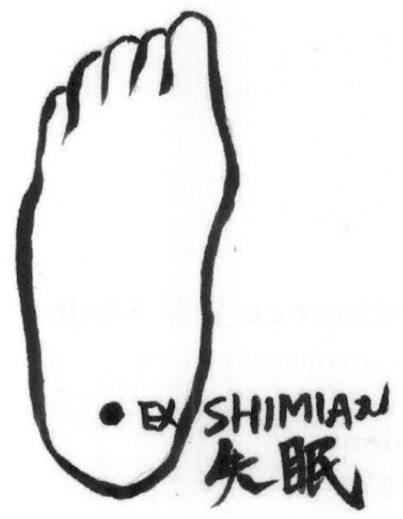

- **Secondary point**
  EX-HN16 (Anmian 安眠)
- Behind the ear, between GB-20 (Fengchi 风池)
  and SJ-17 (Yifeng 翳风).

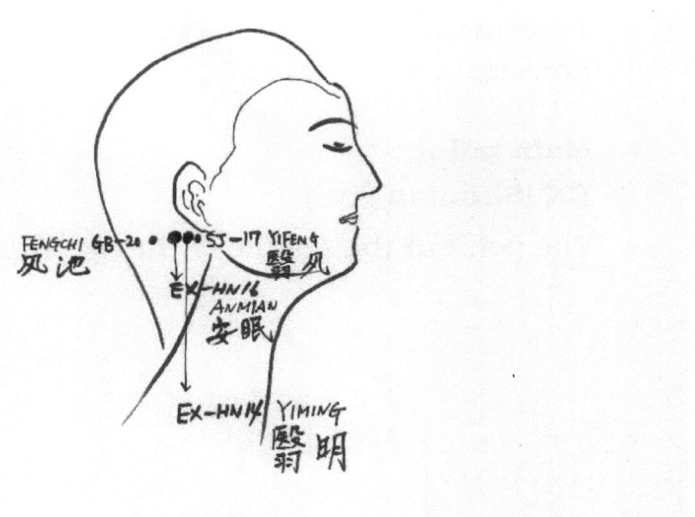

1-21 Incontinence 失禁 Shijin

This refers to involuntary urinary discharge.

- **Treatment**
  Prescription

- **Main point**
  BL-32 (Ciliao 次髎)

- On the sacrum, second posterior sacral
  foramen.

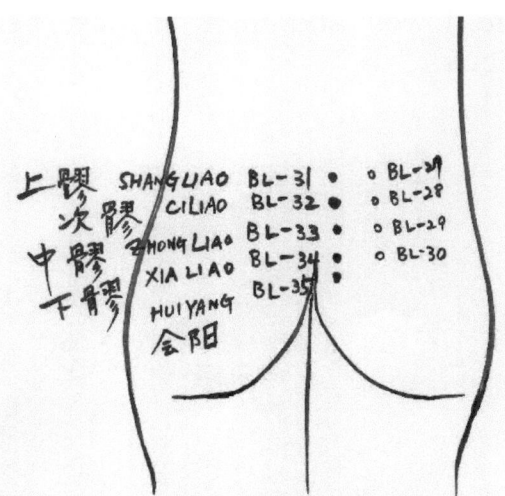

1-22 Impotence 阳痿 Yangwei

It is characterized by the penis inability and erection.
The manifestation shows, dizziness, blurring vision,
listlessness, poor sprit, frequent urination,
weakness knee and lumbar region, insomnia,
palpitation, Heart and Spleen may be involved.

- **Treatment**
  Prescription

- **Main point**
  REN-4 (Guanyuan 关元)
- Front-Mu point of the Small Intestine.
- On the lower abdomen, 3 cun below the umbilicus.

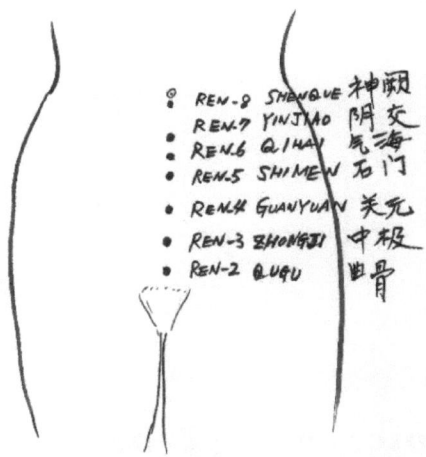

1-23 Indigetion and no appetite 消化不良 Xiaohua buliang

Indigestion is a condition in which food is not properly digested and absorbed in the stomach and intestines due to impaired gastrointestinal motility and insufficient digestive fluids. You may have no appetite because the food in your stomach has not been completely digested.

- **Treatment**
  Prescription

- **Main point**
  ST-36 (Zusanli 足三里)
- He-Sea point of the Stomach channel.
  3 cun inferior to ST-35 (Dubi 犊鼻), one fingerbreadth (middle finger) lateral to the anterior crest of the tibia.

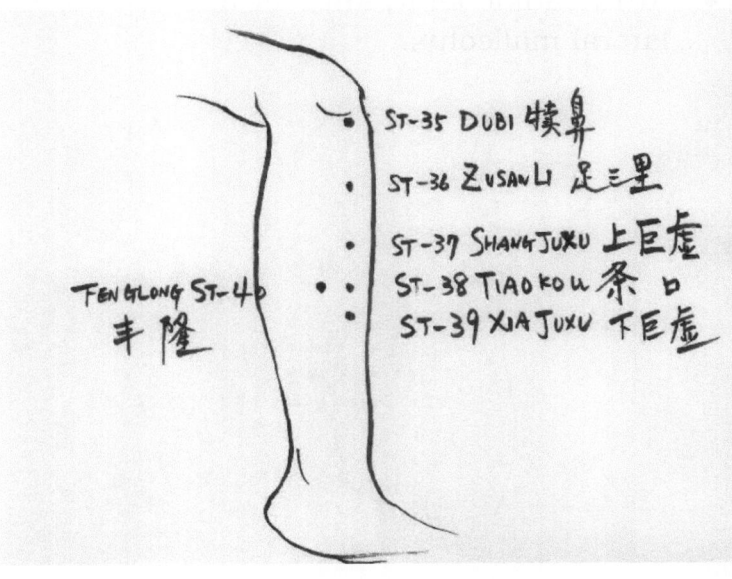

1-24 Intercostal Neuralgia 肋间神经痛 Le jian shenjing tong

This is characterized by pricking pain of the intercostal nerve. Main manifestations are often pain in one or more intercostal spaces.

- **Treatment**
  Prescription

- **Main point**
  GB-40 (Qiuxu 丘墟)
- Yuan-Source point of the Gall Bladder channel.
- At the ankle joint, anterior and inferior to the lateral malleolus.

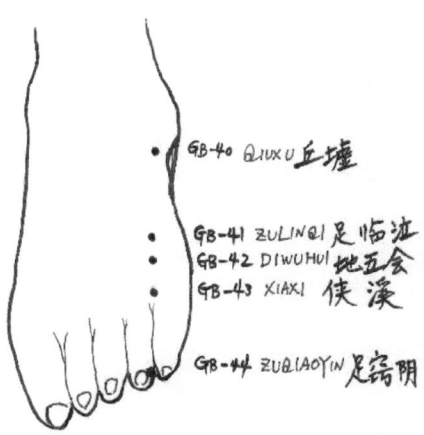

1-25 Lower back pain 下腰痛 Xiayaotong

50 to 60% of lower back pain is caused by muscle fatigue in the back and abdominal muscles.
When looking at the spine from the side, it is normal for it to curve in an S-shape.
If the lumbar vertebrae are not normal, the nerves that come out between the lumbar vertebrae may come into contact with it, then causing pain.

Low back pain occurs often after invasion in pathogenic wind, cold and damp. The pain is characterized by a rapid onset of aching and soreness, stiffness of muscles, limiting extension and flexion of the back. The pain may lead downward to the buttocks and lower extremities that makes the patient feel difficult to bend forward and backward. Pain becomes worse in cloudy and rainy days.

- **Treatment**
  Prescription

- **Main point**
  BL-56 (Chengjin 承筋)
- On the lower leg, 5 cun below BL-40 (Weizhong 委中), in the centre of the belly of gastrocnemius muscle.

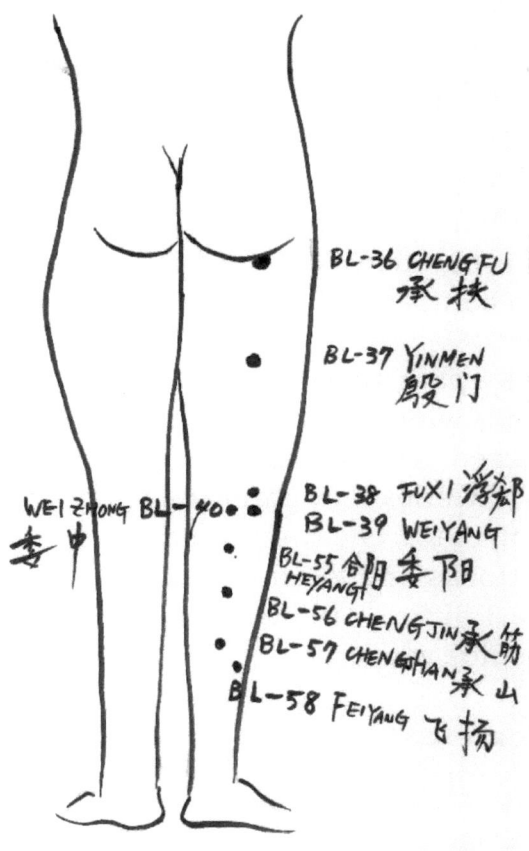

BL-36 CHENGFU 承扶

BL-37 YINMEN 殷门

WEI ZHONG BL-40 委中

BL-38 FUXI 浮郄
BL-39 WEIYANG 委阳

BL-55 合阳
HEYANG

BL-56 CHENGJIN 承筋

BL-57 CHENGSHAN 承山

BL-58 FEIYANG 飞扬

1-26 Periarthritis of Shoulder 肩周炎 Jian zhou yan

Caused by muscle weakness and aging of the shoulder joint. It is a type of aging phenomenon, and is caused by overworked muscles, decreased strength, and aging of the shoulder joint. Apply ice while it is swollen, and then after that to make warm around the shoulder joint. If the pain is severe, rest and then do exercise.

Shoulder pain is named in TCM as frozen shoulder or fifty years old shoulder. The exogenous pathogenic wind, cold and damp overcome patients who are exhausted, overstrained, injured, and while sleeping in the shoulder.

- **Treatment**
  Prescription

- **Main point**
  SJ-13 (Naohui 臑会)
- On the lateral side of the upper arm, on the line connecting the tip of the olecranon and SJ-14 (Jianliao 肩髎), 3 cun below SJ-14 (Jianliao 肩髎).

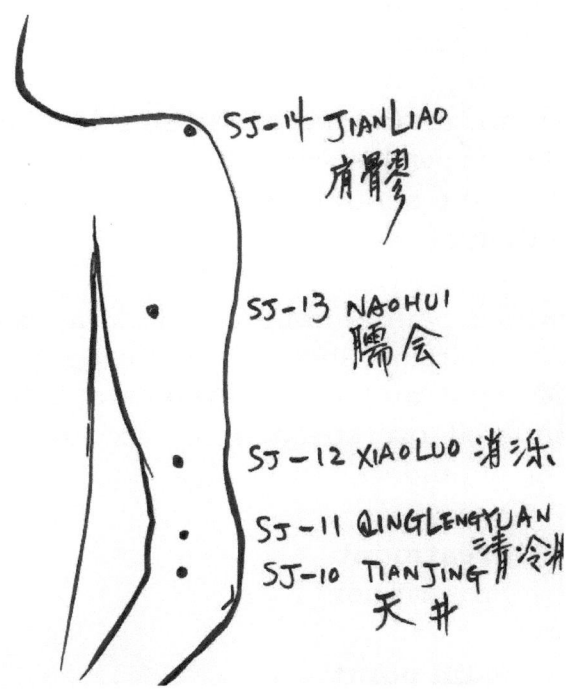

SJ-14 JIANLIAO 肩髎

SJ-13 NAOHUI 臑会

SJ-12 XIAOLUO 消泺

SJ-11 QINGLENGYUAN 清冷渊

SJ-10 TIANJING 天井

- **Secondary point**
  ST-38 (Tiaokou 条口)
- On the lower leg, 8 cun inferior to ST-35 (Dubi 犊鼻), one finger-breadth (middle finger) lateral to the anterior crest of the tibia.

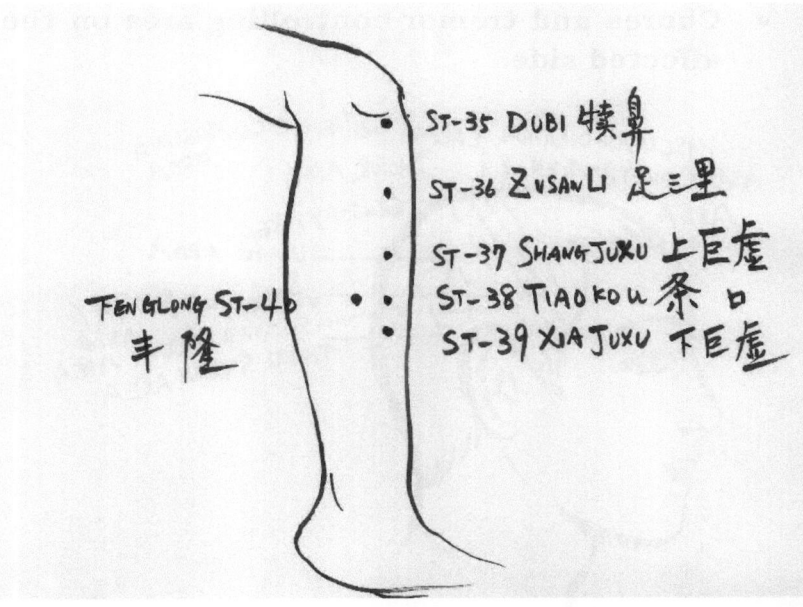

ST-35 DUBI 犊鼻
ST-36 ZUSANLI 足三里
ST-37 SHANGJUXU 上巨虚
ST-38 TIAOKOU 条口
ST-39 XIAJUXU 下巨虚
FENGLONG ST-40 丰隆

1-27 Rheumatic Chorea (involuntary movements) 风湿性舞蹈病 Fengshi xing wudao bing

Weakness and involuntary movement of the limbs. This is limited to limbs on one side of the body. It may be damage to the basal ganglia.

- **Treatment**
  Prescription

- **Chorea and tremor controlling area on the affected side.**

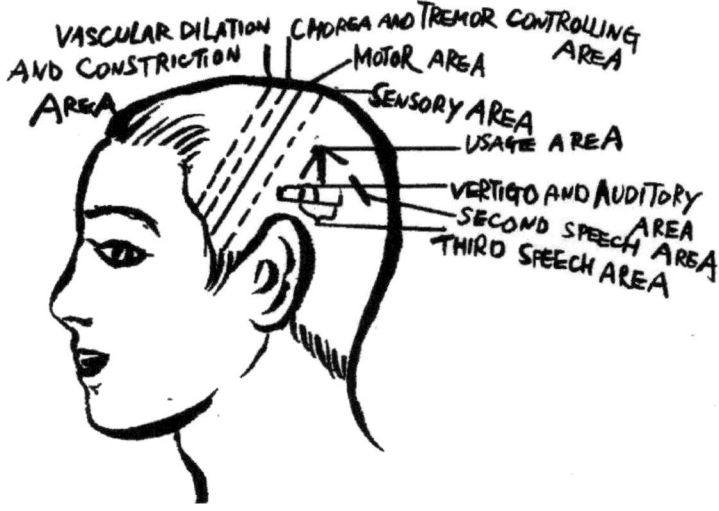

1-28 Retention of Urine 癃闭 Longbi

Manifestations are distention in the lower abdomen, dribbling of urine, pain and distention in lower abdomen.

- **Treatment**
  Prescription

- **Main point**
  REN-3 (Zhongji 中极)
- Front-Mu point of the Bladder.

- On the lower abdomen, 4 cun below the umbilicus.

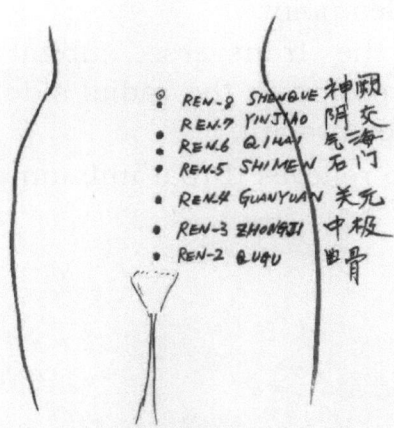

1-29 Sore throat 咽喉肿 Yanhouzhongtong

A sore throat is caused by inflammation of the mucous membranes.

The mucous membrane of the throat has a highly immune system that protects against bacterial infection from the outside air.

These are called tonsils, and they trap bacteria, viruses, dust, etc., and prevent them from entering the lungs and bronchi.

- **Treatment**
  Prescription

- **Main point**
  LU-5 (Chize 尺泽)
- He Sea point
- On the transverse cubital crease, in the depression at the radial side of the tendon of biceps brachii.
- LU-5 relieves throat inflammation and pain.

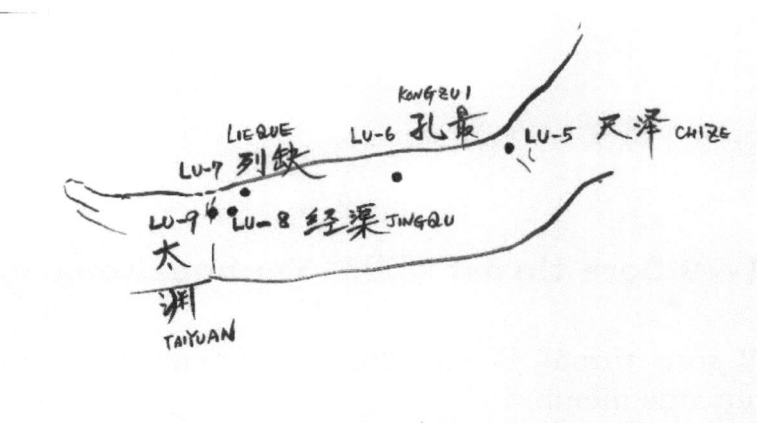

1-30 Schizophrenia 精神分裂症
Jingshenfenliezheng

It often occurs in young adults, and generally, genetic and environmental factors are considered, but it needs many years for studies and research.

It characterized by incoherence of thinking, delusion, hallucination, mania, insomnia, not sleep whole night, depression, dry skin, inactivity etc.

- **Treatment**
  Prescription

- **Main point**
  DU-16 (Fengfu 风府)
- Point of the Sea of Marrow.
- On the neck, 1cun above the midpoint of the posterior hairline, below the external occipital protuberance.

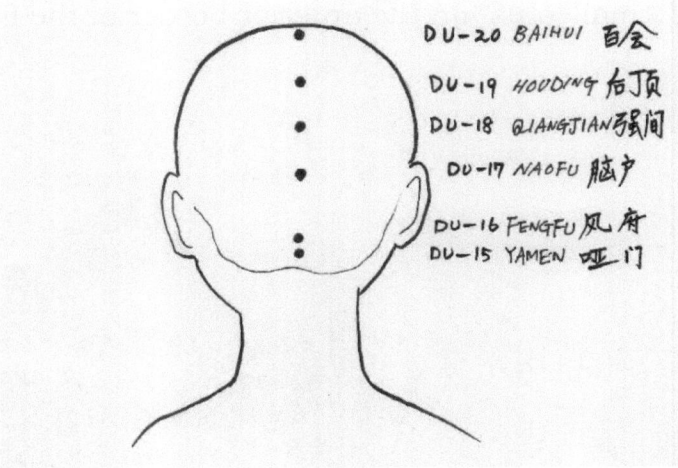

1-31 Stiff Neck 落枕 Laozhen

It is caused by exogenous pathogenic wind and cold and also while sleeping. Some cases may have the pain spread to the shoulder of the affected side, and it aggravate by movement of the neck.

- **Treatment**
  Prescription

- **Main point**
  GB-39 (Xuanzhong 悬钟)

- On the lateral side of the lower leg, 3 cun superior to the prominence of the lateral malleolus, on the anterior border of the fibula.

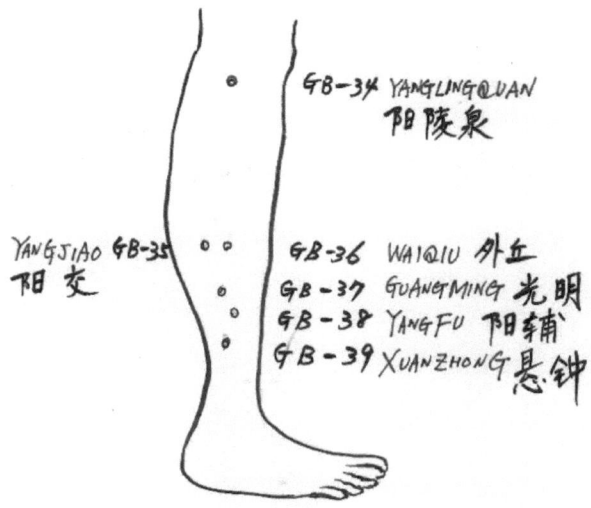

GB-34 YANGLINGQUAN 阳陵泉

YANGJIAO GB-35 阳交

GB-36 WAIQIU 外丘
GB-37 GUANGMING 光明
GB-38 YANGFU 阳辅
GB-39 XUANZHONG 悬钟

- **combined point**
  SI-3 (Houxi 后溪)
- When a loose fist is made, the point on the ulnar side of the hand, at the end of the transverse crease proximal to the fifth metacarpophalangeal joint.

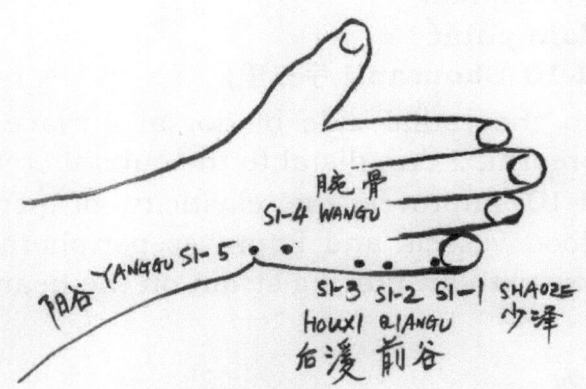

1-32 Shoulder pain 肩痛 Jiantong

Stiff shoulders and pain refer to symptoms such as muscle tension, discomfort, and dull pain from the neck to the shoulders.

Shoulder pain is named in TCM as frozen shoulder or fifty years old shoulder. The exogenous pathogenic wind, cold and damp overcome patients who are exhausted, overstrained, injured, and while sleeping in the shoulder.

The most important thing is to improve blood flow. By improving blood flow, nutrients and oxygen are carried in, and waste products are carried away, which relieves stiffness.

- **Treatment**
  Prescription
- **Main point**
  LI-10 (Shousanli 手三里)
- On the radial side of dorsal surface of the forearm, 2 cun distal to the cubital crease.
- LI-10 improves the elasticity of peripheral blood vessels and improves peripheral blood flow without putting strain on the heart.

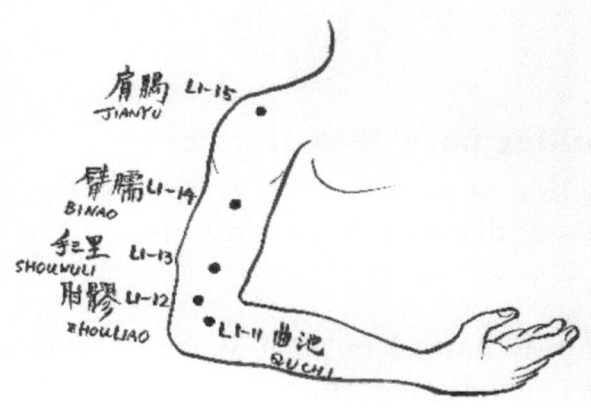

- **Secondary point
  Li-15 (Jianyu 肩髃)**
- On the shoulder, in the depression anterior border of the acromioclavicular point.

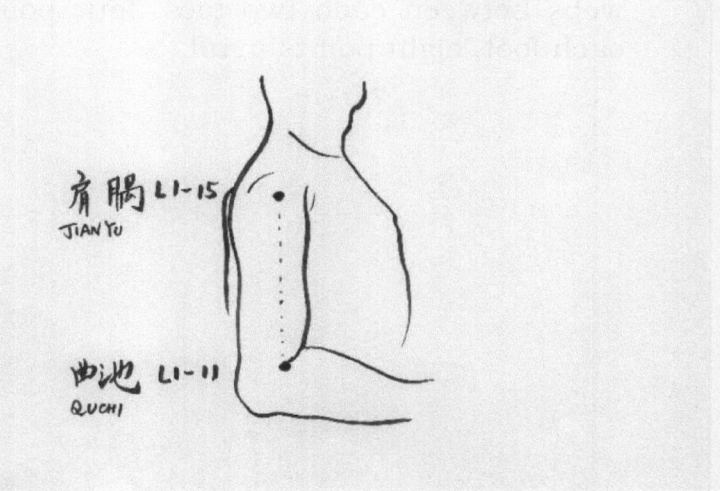

1-33 Sprain Ankle 扭伤脚踝 Niushang jiaohuai

Sprains tend to occur in the ankle. A sprain is caused by excessive joint movement, which applies excessive force from the outside to the membranes and ligaments surrounding the joint, even though the joint remains in its normal position.

- **Treatment**
  Prescription
- **Main point**
  EX-LE9 (Bafeng 八风)
- On the dorsum of the foot, at the margin of the webs between each two toes, four points on each foot, eight points in all.

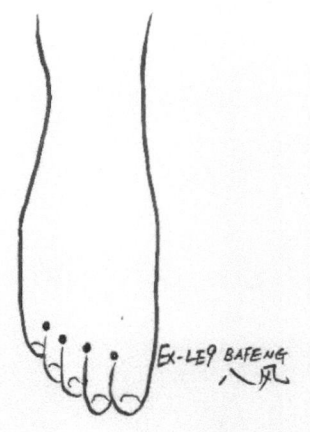

- **Secondary point**
  Ashi point

1-34 Seminal Emission 遗精 Yijing

This refers to nocturnal emission and the involuntary emission. Nocturnal emission may be with dreams, dizziness, palpitation, listlessness, lassitude, yellow urine, red tongue, thready rapid pulse.

Involuntary Emission may be with frequent mission, pallor complexion, listlessness, soreness in the lumbar region, emaciation, pale tongue, deep thready pulse.

- **Treatment**
  Prescription

- **Main point**
  REN-3 (Zhongji 中极)
- Front-Mu point of the Bladder.
- On the lower abdomen, 4 cun below the umbilicus.

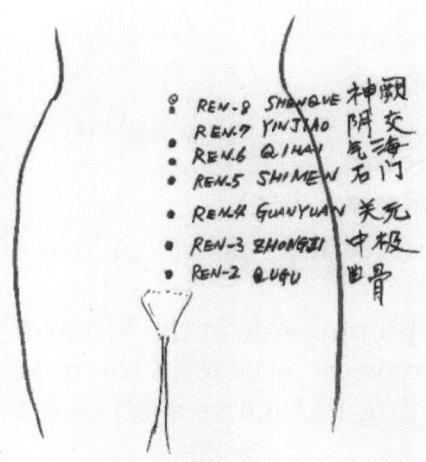

1-35 Vomiting 呕吐 Outu

1. This is characterized by epigastric distention, casting up of sour tastes, belching, abdominal pain, foul gas, constipation, greasy tongue coating, slippery pulse.

2. Invasion of Stomach by Liver Qi
   This is characterized by vomiting, acid regurgitation, frequent belching, distention in the hypochondriac region, thin greasy tongue coating, wiry pulse.

3. Weakness of Stomach and Spleen
   Sallow complexion, lack of appetite, loose stools, pale, sticky tongue, weak soft pulse.

- **Treatment**
  Prescription

- **Main point**
  P-6 (Neiguan 内关)
- Luo-Connecting point of the Pericardium channel.
- On the palmar side of the forearm, 2 cun above the transverse crease of the wrist, on the line connecting P-3 (Quze 曲泽) and P-7 (Daling 大

陵), between the tendons of palmaris longus and flexor carpi radialis.

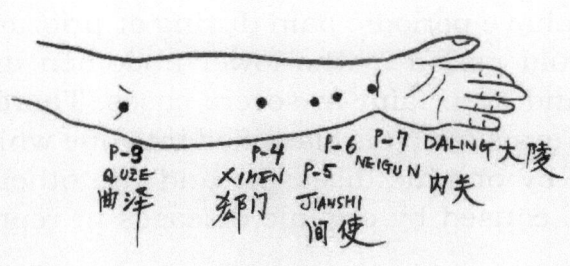

1-36 Tennis Elbow 网球肘 Wangqiu zhou

It manifests itself in pain of the tendon of forearm extensors, on the lateral side of the elbow joint. It can radiate to shoulder and wrist, and the affected arm feels sore and weak.

- **Treatment**
  Prescription

- **Main point**
  Ashi point

Chapter 2 Gynecology

2-1 Dysmenorrhea (痛经 Tongjing)

Women have periodic pain during or prior to or after menstrual period in the lower abdomen and lower back, and even faint in severe cases. There are two main groups which is classified into one which is not caused by organic diseases, and the other refer to the one caused by organic diseases in reproductive system.

- **Treatment**
  Prescription

- **Main point**
  EX-B8 (Shiqizhui 十七椎)
- On the lower back, the posterior midline below the spinous process of the fifth lumbar vertebra.

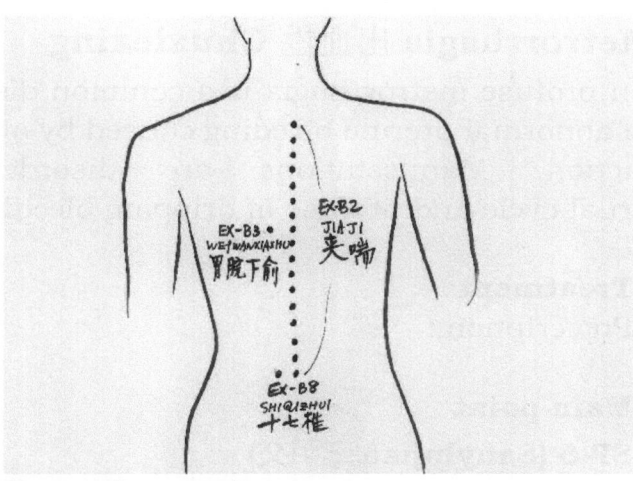

- **Secondary point**

SP-6 (Sanyinjiao 三阴交)

- 3 cun directly above the tip of medial malleolus, in the depression near the posterior border of the tibia.

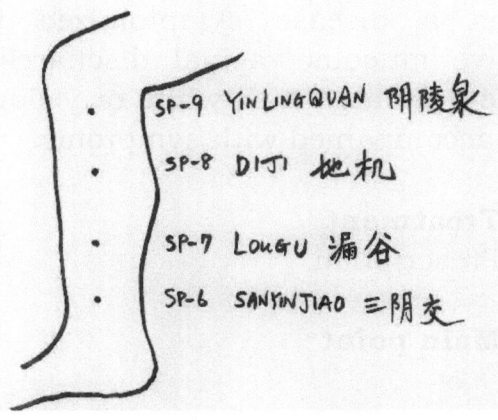

2-2 Metrorrhagia 出血性 Chuxiexing

Sudden profuse metrorrhagia is a common disease. It is an abnormal uterine bleeding caused by ovarian dysfunction. Manifestations are disorder of menstrual cycle and profuse of dripping bleeding.

- **Treatment**
  Prescription

- **Main point**
  SP-6 (Sanyinjiao 三阴交)
- 3 cun directly above the tip of medial malleolus, in the depression near the posterior border of the tibia.

2-3 Leukorrhagia 带下 Daixia

This is a disease symptomized by persistent excessive mucous vaginal discharge. It refers to profuse discharge with white or yellow, quality and smell, accompanied with symptoms.

- **Treatment**
  Prescription

- **Main point**

- **REN-6 (Qihai 气海)**
- Sea of Qi.
- On the lower abdomen, 1.5 cun below the umbilicus.

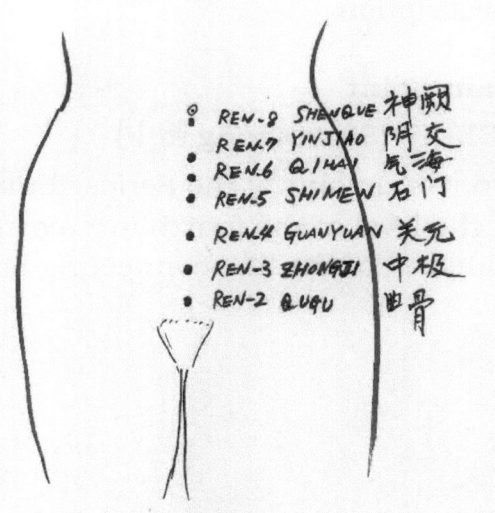

- **Secondary point**
- **SP-6 (Sanyinjiao 三阴交)**
- 3 cun directly above the tip of medial malleolus, in the depression near the posterior border of the tibia.

2-4 Lactation deficiency 乳汁少 Ruzhishao

It is characterized by scanty or absence of milk after childbirth or decrease in quantity during lactation.

- **Treatment**
  Prescription

- **Main point**
  REN-17 (Shanzhong 膻中)
- Front-Mu point of the Pericardium.
- At the level of the fourth intercostal space, the midpoint of the line connecting both nipples.

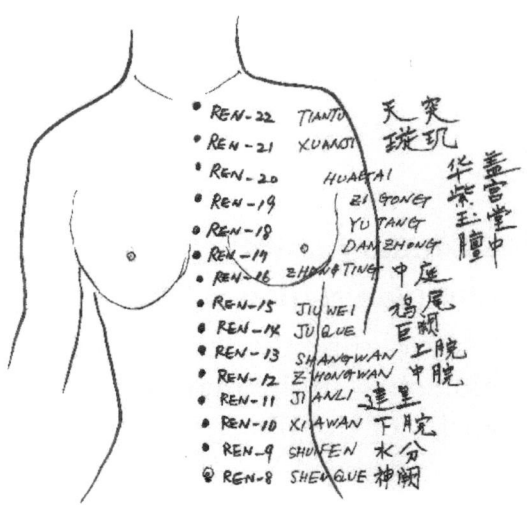

2-5 Postpartum retention of Urine 产后尿潴留 Chanhou niao zhuliu

This is due to difficult labor resulting in large amounts of urine accumulated in the bladder. It characterized by blockage of urine, distension and fullness in the lower abdomen.

- **Treatment**
  Prescription
- **Main point**
  REN-8 (Shenque 神阙)
- In the centre of the umbilicus.

2-6 Postpartum complications 产后并发症 Chanhou bingfa zheng

The mother becomes weak, tired, angry after delivery, and leads to insomnia.

- **Treatment**
  Prescription

- **Main point**
  DU-20 (Baihui 白会)
- Point of the Sea of Marrow.

- On the midline of the head, 5 cun above the midpoint of the anterior hairline, at the midpoint connecting the apexes of both ears.

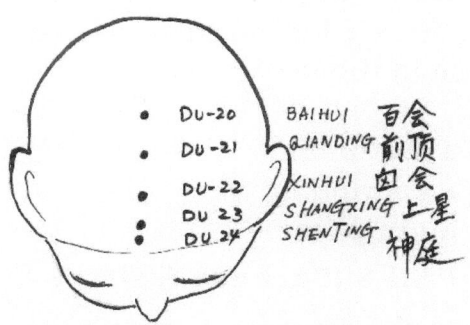

2-7 Acute Mastadenitis 急性乳腺炎
Jíxìng rǔxiàn yán

This is suppurative inflammation of the mammary gland, and by the infection of bacteria. That invades the breast by the splitting of the nipple or the retention of milk.

- **Treatment**
  Prescription

- **Main point**
  GB-21 (Jianjing 肩井)

- On the shoulder, directly above the nipple, midway between DU-14(Dazhui 大椎) and the tip of the acromion.

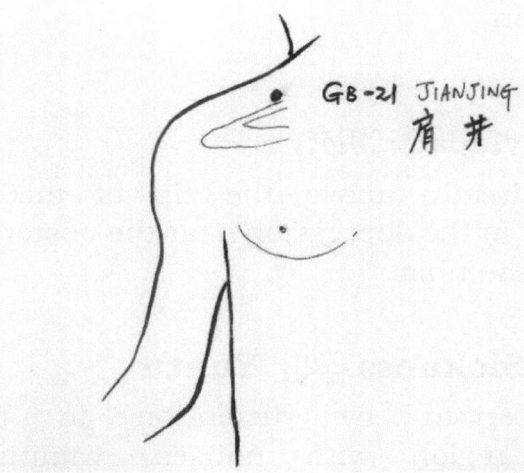

2-8 Irregular menstruation 月经不调 Yuejingbutiao

Irregular menstruation is when the interval between periods is long or short. The other thing is that the amount of menstruation itself may be heavy or small, and the period may be 3 days or 10 days.

The function of the ovaries determines the menstrual rhythm. The brain command system controls the ovaries. If there is an abnormality in any part of this mechanism, menstrual irregularities will occur.

- **Treatment**
  Prescription

- **Main point**
  SP-6 (Sanyinjiao 三阴交)
  - 3 cun directly above the tip of medial malleolus, in the depression near the posterior border of the tibia.

2-9 Morning Sickness 孕吐 Yuntu

It is characterized by distention in the hypochondriac region with nausea, vomiting, dizziness may take place right after food intake or smell of food.

- **Treatment**
  Prescription

- **Main point**
  Shenmen (神门) ear acupuncture

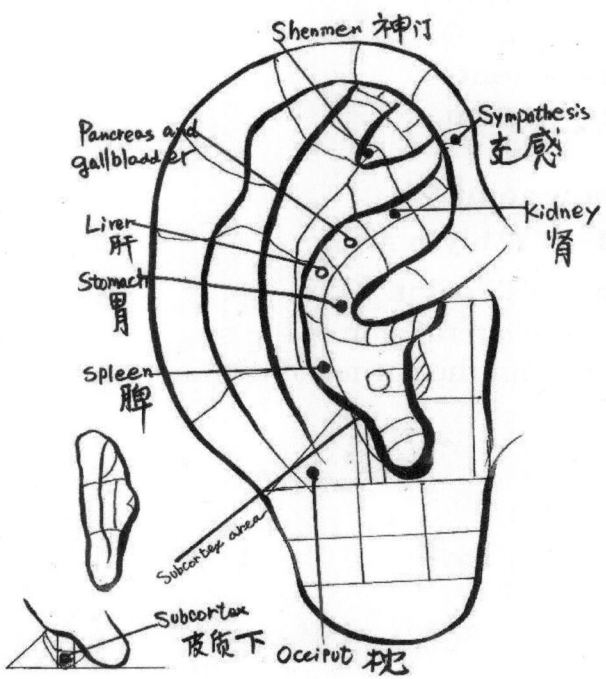

Shenmen 神门
Sympathesis 交感
Pancreas and gallbladder
Kidney 肾
Liver 肝
Stomach 胃
Spleen 脾
Subcortex area
Subcortex 皮质下
Occiput 枕

2-10 Malposition of Fetus 胎位不正
Taiweibuzheng

Malposition of Fetus means that the fetus is in an abnormal position in the uterus after thirty weeks of pregnancy. It is often seen in multipara or pregnant women who have laxity of the abdominal wall.

- **Treatment**
  Prescription

- **Main point**
  BL-67 (Zhiyin 至阴)

- Jing-Well point.
- On the lateral side of the small toe, about 0.1 cun from the corner of the nail.

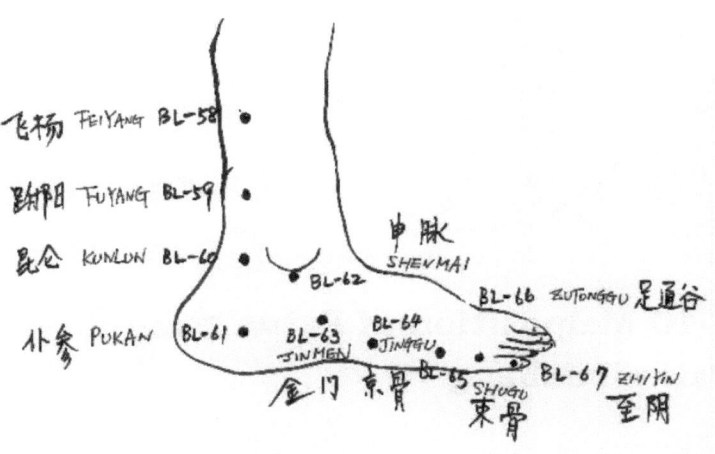

Chapter 3 Surgical & Dermatological Disease

3-1 Acne 痤疮 Cuochuang

Acne is most cases on face, which may release white bodies upon squeezing. This follows by the formation of small pustules with tidal feverish, itching and pain sensation. It often occurs in adolescence.

- **Treatment**
  Prescription

- **Main point**
  DU-14 (Dazhui 大椎)
- Point of the Sea of Qi.
- Meeting point of the Governing vessel with Six Yang channel.
- At the level of the shoulder, in the depression below the spinous process of the seventh cervical vertebra.

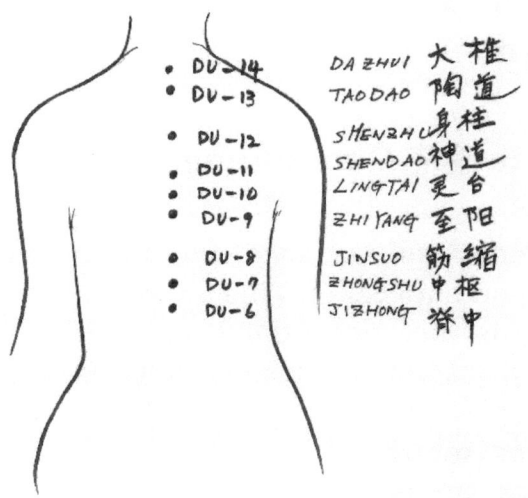

3-2 Eczema 湿疹 Shizhen

It is a allergic inflammatory dermatosis. It is divided into acute and chronic types.

Acute is characterized by a rapid onset of erythema. The clusters and flakes may break by scratching, and it may turn into severe itching sensation.

Chronic type is that after repeated attacking eczema for a long time, it may be caused blood deficiency. The manifestations are roughness of skin.

- **Treatment**
Prescription

- **Main point**
DU-14 (Dazhui 大椎)
- Point of the Sea of Qi.
- Meeting point of the Governing vessel with Six Yang channel.
- At the level of the shoulder, in the depression below the spinous process of the seventh cervical vertebra.

3-3 Psoriasis 银屑病 Yinxiebing

t refers to a chronic skin condition characterized by repeated scaled dermatosis, and have some dry silver, white scales covered.

- **Treatment**
Prescription

- **Main point**
LI-11 (Quchi 曲池)
- He-Sea point.
- In the depression at the lateral end of the transverse cubital crease.

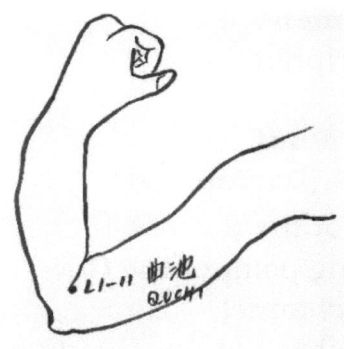

- **Ear acupuncture**

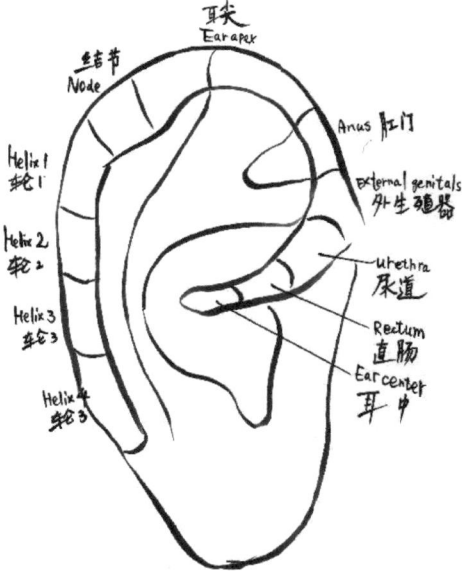

Ear apex (erjian 耳尖)

- Ear apex point is located at the upper tip auricle and superior to helix when folded towards tragus.

3-4 Urticaria 荨麻疹 Xunmazhen

It is abrupt onset with itching flat-topped wheals of various size on the skin. In TCM, it calls Wind Wheal.

The manifestations are the appearance of wheals over the skin with sudden onset and rapid disappearance, and there is no trace after recovery. There is severe itching and red rashes on the affected part.

- **Treatment**
  Prescription

- **Main point**
  REN-8 (Shenque 神阙)
- In the centre of the umbilicus.

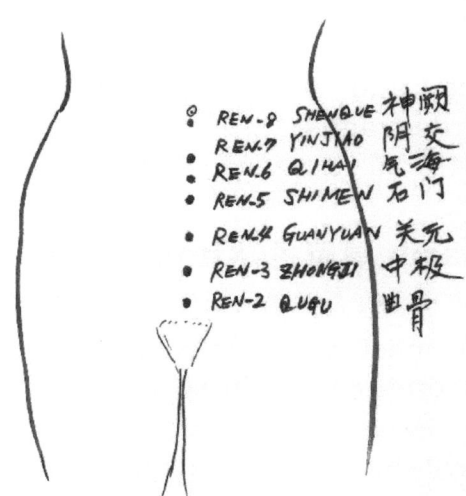

3-5 Hemorrhoids 痔疮 Zhichuang

There are two sphincters in the anus: an outer and an inner sphincter. When you strain to defecate, the tip of the intestine protrudes from the anus, and the sphincter muscle tightens on it, causing congestion and wart-like formations. Hemorrhoids are those that tear and bleed when you defecate. Both are very painful.

If you sit for a long time or stay in a cold place, the blood flow around your intestines and buttocks becomes poor, and your muscles become weaker. On the other hand, if the blood flow around the buttocks is good, the intestines will be elastic, warts will not form, and there will be no tears.

- **Treatment**
  Priscriptions
- **Main point**

  LU-6 (Kongzui 孔最)

- Xi-Cleft point
- On the medial border of the radius, along the line connection LU-5, 5 cun below. 7 cun above the LU-9.
- LU-6 has a hemostatic effect and effective point for hemorrhoids.

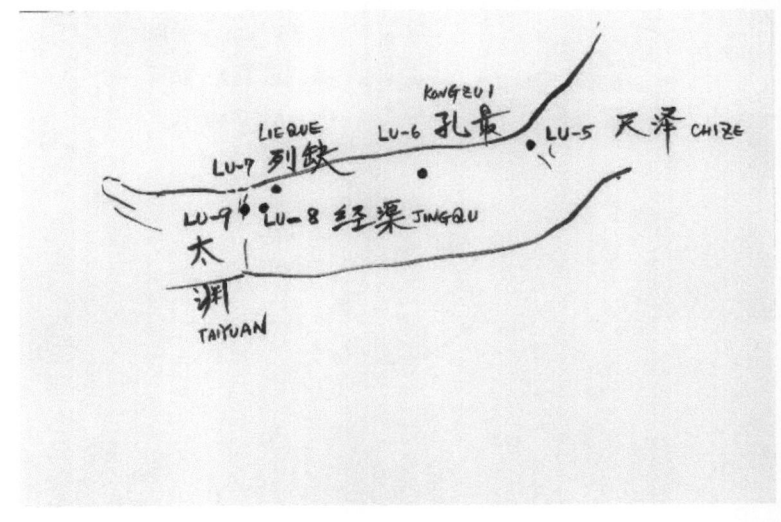

- **Secondary point**
  ST-37 (Shangjuxu 上巨虚)
- Lower He-Sea point of the Large Intestine.
- On the lower leg, 6 cun inferior to ST-35 (Dubi 犊鼻), one finger- breadth (middle finger) lateral to the anterior crest of the tibia.

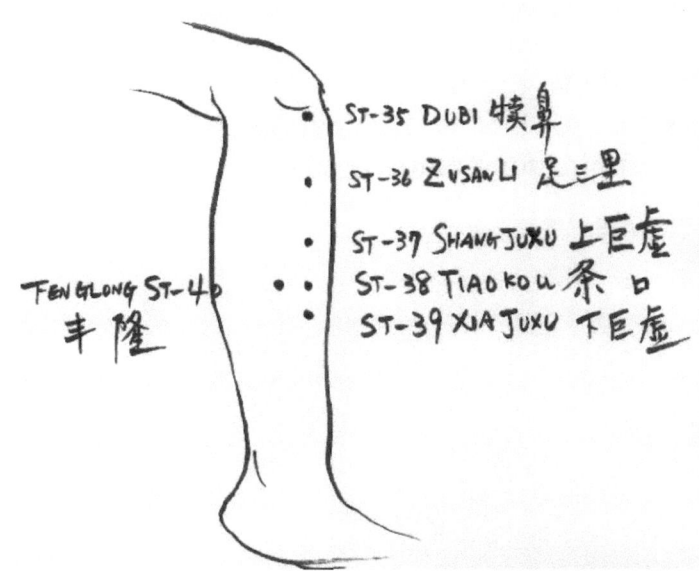

ST-35 DUBI 犊鼻

ST-36 ZUSANLI 足三里

ST-37 SHANGJUXU 上巨虚

ST-38 TIAOKOU 条口

ST-39 XIAJUXU 下巨虚

FENGLONG ST-40 丰隆

3-6 Ureterolithiasis 输尿管结石
Shuniaoguan jieshi

This is a common disease in the urinary system, f. ex. Calculus of the kidney, ureteral calculus, urethral calxulus and vesical calculus.

- **Treatment**
  Priscriptions

- **Main point**
  KI-3 (Taixi 太溪)
- Yuan-Source of the Kidney channel.
- On the medial malleolus, in the depression between the prominence of the medial malleolus and the Achilles tendon.

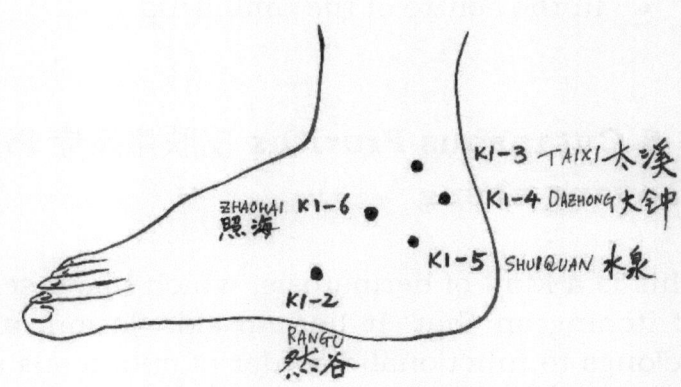

3-7 Prostatitis 前列腺炎 Manxing qianliexian yan

This is a disease of the urinary system in young and middle-aged male patients. The disease which may be infection of acute prostatitis, posterior urethritis, infection of the upper respiratory tract or mouth cavity. The common pathogens are streptococcus, colibacillus, and staphylococcus. This may be caused by injury of the perineum, excessive alcoholic intaking, and excessive sexual intercourses.

- **Treatment**
  Prescription

- **Main point**
  REN-8 (Shenque 神阙)
- In the centre of the umbilicus.

3-8 Cutaneous Pruritus 皮肤瘙痒症 Pifu saoyang zheng

This is a kind of dermatosis, which has a sensation of itching on that. It has no skin lesion, and this belongs to functional disorder of cutaneous sensory nerve.

- **Treatment**
Prescriptions

- **Main point**
KI-9 (Zhubin 筑宾)
- On the medial border of the lower leg, 5 cun superior to KI-3 (Taixi 太溪), on the line connecting KI-3 (Taixi 太溪) and KI-10 (Yingu 阴谷).

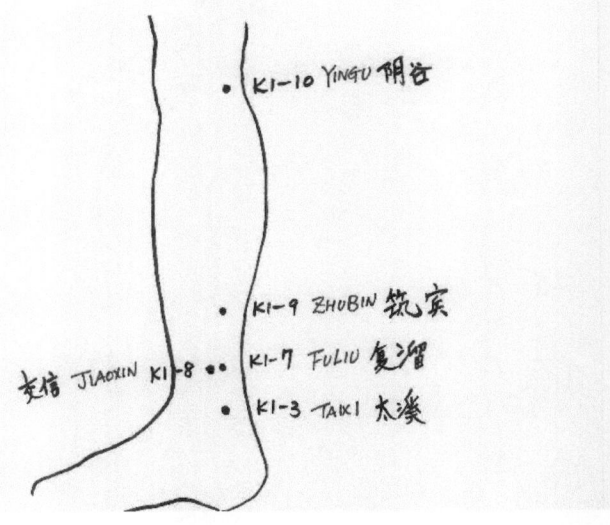

- **Secondary point**
- **SP-10 (Xuehai 血海)**

- Sea of Blood.
- When the knee is flexed, 2 cun above medial border of the patella, directly above SP-9 (Yinlingquan 阴陵泉).
- When the knee is flexed, put the palm on the upper border of the patella with four fingers directed upward, and the thumb forming an angle of 45 degrees with the index finger. The point is where the tip of the thumb.

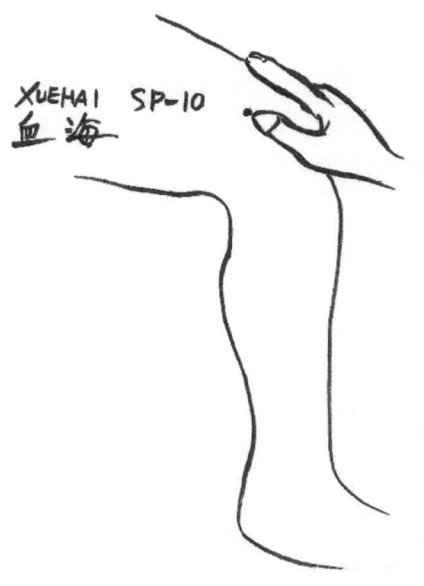

XUEHAI SP-10

血海

3-9 Cholelithiasis (the formations of Gallstones) 胆石症 Danshi zheng

This is affected by cholecystitis and inflammation, and stones are found at the same time. It may cause, flatulence, cholecystitis, obstructive jaundice, biliary colic. They may attack of fever, upper abdominal pain. This is a common surgical disease.

- **Treatment**
  Prescription
- **Main point**
  BL-19 (Danshu 胆俞)

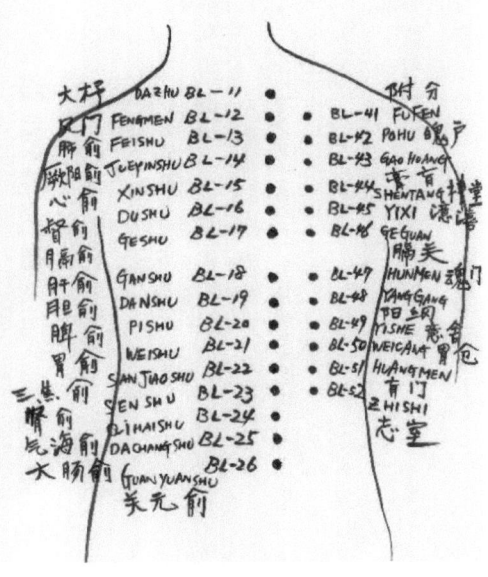

- Back-Shu point of the Gall Bladder.
- On the back, below the spinous process of the tenth thoracic vertebra (T10), 1.5 cun lateral to the posterior midline.

- **Secondary point
  REN-8 (Shenque 神阙)**
- In the centre of the umbilicus.

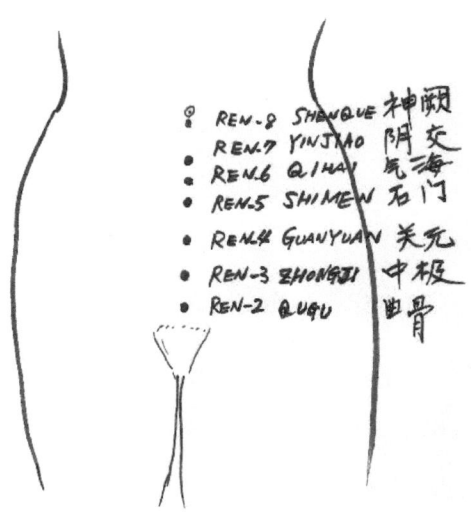

Chapter 4 Pediatric Diseases

4-1 Mumps 腮腺炎 Saixian yan

It is acute infection disease, caused by the mumps virus. It is characterized by swelling and pain of the parotid gland.

- **Treatment**
  Priscriptions

- **Main point**
  SJ-20 (Jiaosun 角孙)
- Directly above the ear apex, within the hair line.

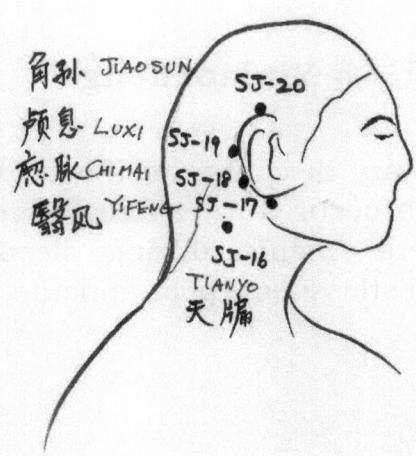

4-2 Infantile Diarrhea 小儿腹泻 **Xiaoerfuxie**

It is a common pediatric disease, mainly manifested by frequent bowel movement, watery feces. It may occur in any season, but more often occurs in summer and autumn. Acute diarrhea may be with improper intake, bacterial infection, or viral infection.

- **Treatment**
  Priscriptions

- **Main point**
  REN-8 (Shenque 神阙)
- In the centre of the umbilicus.

4-3 Enureasis 遗尿症 **Yiniaozheng**

It refers to involuntary discharge of the urine of a child. It happens to occur during sleep. It may be happened in several nights during sleep. The manifestations are listlessness, poor appetite.

- **Treatment**
  Prescription

- **Main point**
  BL-23 (Shenshu 肾俞)
- Back-Shu point of the Kidneys.
- On the lower back, below the spinous process of the second lumbar vertebra (L2), 1.5 cun lateral to the posterior midline.

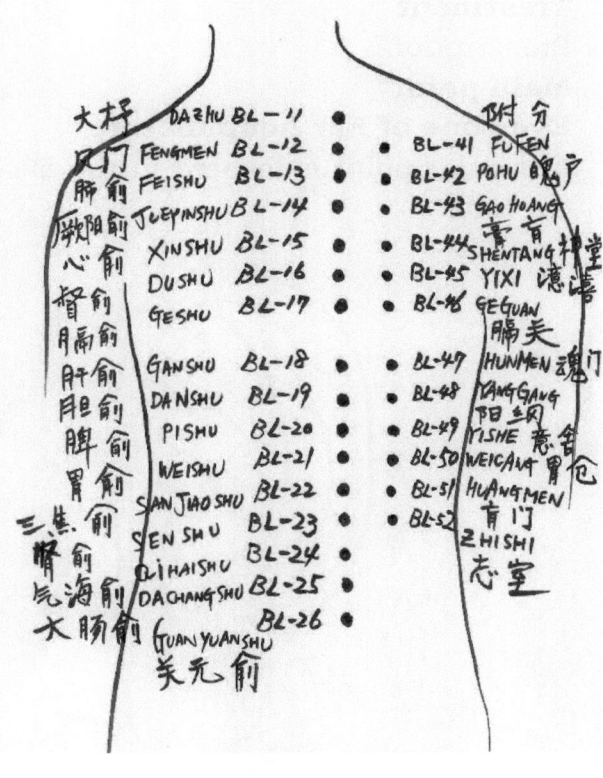

Chapter 5 Diseases of Eyes, Ears, Nose and Throat

5-1 Myopia (Jinshi 近视)

It is characterized in that the eyes can see near objects but not distant.

- **Treatment**
  Prescription
- **Main point**
  Eye zone of Ear Acupuncture
- Auricular point is located in the 5th section of ear lobe.

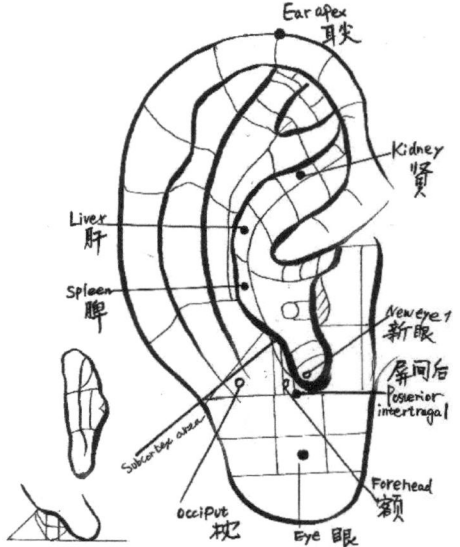

5-2 Dacryorrhea 泪溢 Leiyi

This means tearing, which is caused by hyperactive function of lacrimal secretion.

1. Heat tear

It is due to fire and characterized by the running of hot tears against the wind. It caused by accumulation of heat in the Liver and invasion of exogenous pathogenic wind, and it may be exposed Yin deficiency. It is manifested run of hot teas, reddened, swollen eyes, burning pain.

2. Cold tear

The manifestations show lacrimation, thinness of the tears without hot feeling, but it runs of tears to the cheek in some cases.

- **Treatment**
  Prescription

- **Main point**
  EX-HN5 (Taiyang 太阳)
- At the temporal part of the head, in the depression 1 cun posterior to the midpoint between the lateral end of the eyebrow and the outer canthus of the eye.

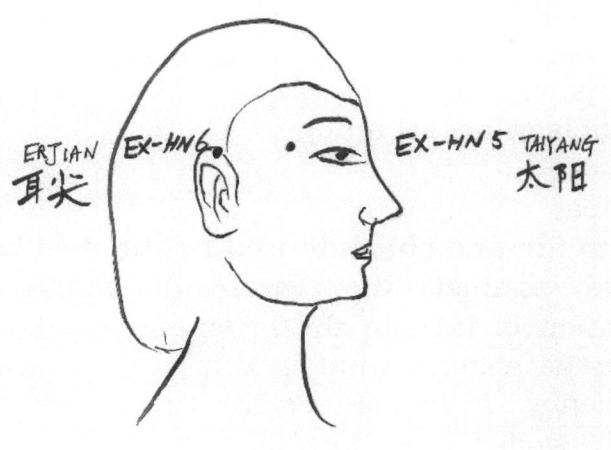

5-3 Optic Atrophy 视神经萎
Shishenjingweisuo

This is a chronic eye disorder marked by gradual degeneration of vision.

- **Treatment**
  Prescription

- **Main point**
  EX-UE6 (Xiaogukong 小骨空)

- On the dorsal side of the little finger, at the midpoint of the proximal interphalangeal joint.

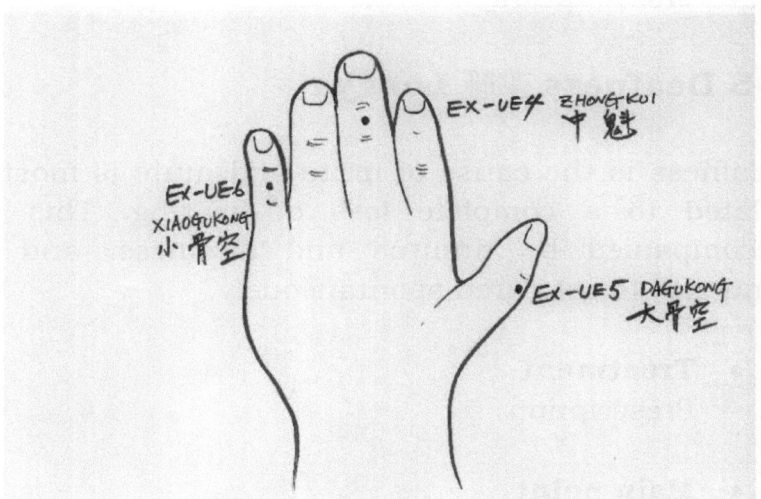

5-4 Stye 麦粒肿 Mailizhong

It refers to the inflammatory furuncle of the sebaceous gland of the eyelid, and often occurs among young people. The manifestations are itching, redness and pain.

- **Treatment**
  Prescription
- **Main point**

EX-UE6 (Xiaogukong 小骨空)

- On the dorsal side of the little finger, at the midpoint of the proximal interphalangeal joint.
- **Moxibustion**

5-5 Deafness 聋哑 Longya

Deafness is the cause of mute and mute is mostly related to a complete loss of hearing. This is accompanied by tinnitus and dizziness, and a tendency to get cured spontaneously.

- **Treatment**
  Prescription

- **Main point**
  SI-19 (Tinggong 听宫)
- In the depression formed when the mouth is open. Anterior to the tragus and posterior to the condyloid process of the mandible.

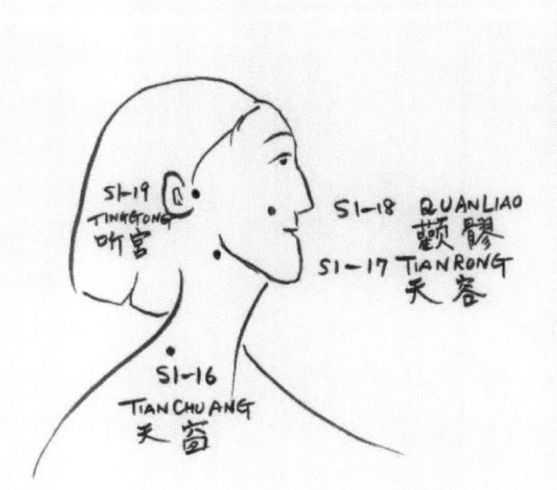

5-6 Tinnitus 耳鸣 Erming

Tinnitus is characterized by continuous ringing sound in the ears.

- **Treatment**
  Prescription
- **Main point**
  SJ-2 (Yemen 液门)
- When the fist is clenched, between the ring and little fingers, proximal to the margin of the web.

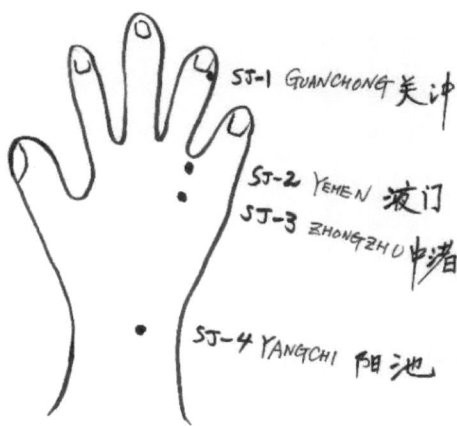

SJ-1 GUANCHONG 关冲

SJ-2 YEMEN 液门
SJ-3 ZHONGZHU 中渚

SJ-4 YANGCHI 阳池

5-7 Rhinitis 鼻炎 Biyan

This is by nasal obstruction and nasal secretion.
This is induced by the exogenous Wind-Cold or Wind-Heat, improper diet, and the manifestations are nasal secretion of thick and yellow mucosa.

- **Treatment**
  Prescription

- **Main point**
  LI 20 (Yingxiang 迎香)
- In the naso-labial groove, at the level of the midpoint of the ala nasi.

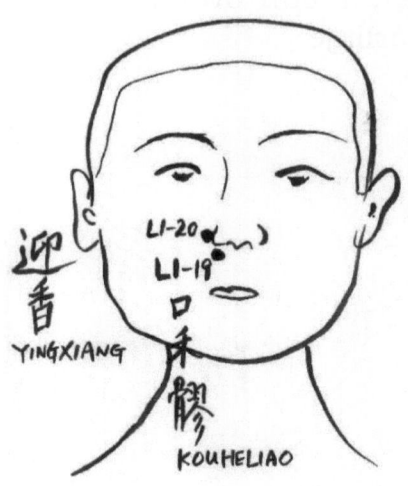

迎
香
YINGXIANG

LI-20
LI-19
口
禾
髎
KOUHELIAO

5-8 Epistaxis 鼻衄 Binü

Epistaxis means nose bleeds, which can be caused by mycteric or general diseases. The naso-nasopharyngeal plexus at the end of the inferior nasal meatus is also an area where nosebleed is apt to occur.

- **Treatment**
  Prescription

- **Main point**
  DU-23 (Shangxing 上星)

- På hovedet, 1 cun over midtpunktet på den forreste hårlinje.

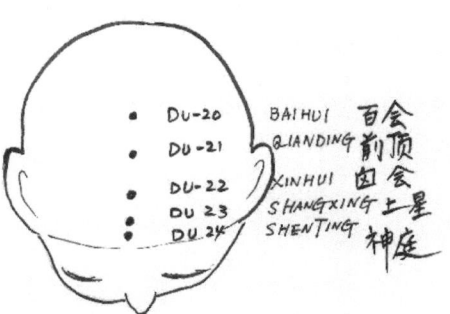

5-9 Tonsillitis 扁桃体炎 Biantaotiyan

It is caused by inflammation by the invasion of streptococcus and staphylococcus. The symptom is marked by swelling, pain, fever, headache, sore throat which is aggravated when swallowing.

- **Treatment**
  Prescription

- **Main point**
  LU-11 (Shaoshang 少商)
- Jing-Well point.

- On the radial side of the thumb, 0.1 cun from the corner of the nail.

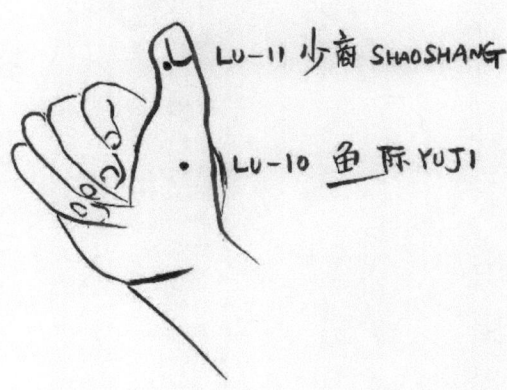

5-10 Plum Throat 梅子喉咙 Meizi houlong

Plum throat is, as if the throat were stuck by a piece of plum. The symptom is dry cough and repeated empty swallowing, dry cough, feel itching.

- **Treatment**
  Prescription

- **Main point**
  REN-22 (Tiantu 天突)

- On the neck, in the centre of the suprasternal fossa.

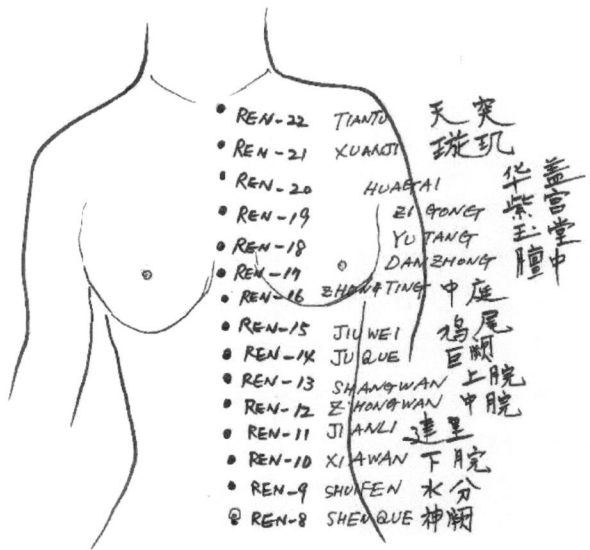

5-11 Ulcer in the mouth 口腔溃疡

Kouqiang kuiyang

This is a kind of scattered small ulcer in the mucous membrane of the mouth.

- **Treatment**
  Prescription

- **Main point**
  REN-8 (Shenque 神阙)

- In the centre of the umbilicus.

5-12 Stuffy Nose 鼻塞 Bise

Nasal congestion can come from a cold or from empyema.

A condition in which the nasal passages are clogged with nasal discharge, which can be a runny nose, mucous nasal discharge, or hardened nasal discharge. It is normal for mucus to come out of nose, so if it let it drain smoothly, it won't get stuck in the nasal passages.

- **Treatment**
  Prescription

- **Main point**
  HT-3 (Shaohai 少海)
- He-Sea point of the Heart channel.
- When the elbow is flexed, at the midpoint of the line jointing the medial end of the transverse cubital crease.

- HT-3 improves blood flow in the nose and has the effect of smoothing out nasal secretions. HT-3 is Acu point with colds and health, regulating immune function.

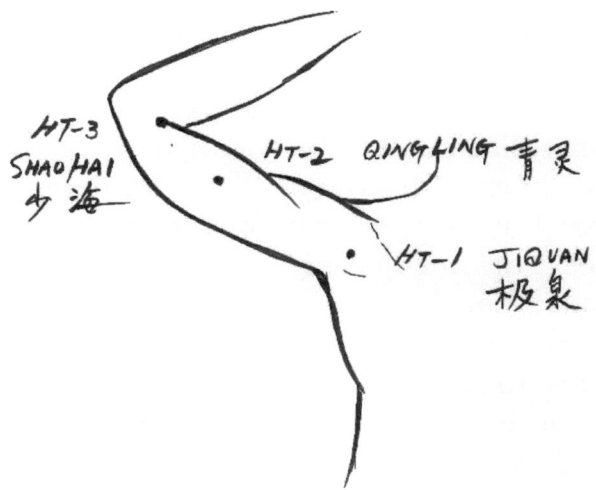

5-13 Nosebleed 鼻血 Bixie

Nosebleeds occur not only due to serious illnesses, but also when you have a hot flash, cold, or blow your nose, nosebleeds tend to occur about 1cm deep from inside of the nose, where capillaries are densely at the shallow surface, so even a slight injury will cause bleeding.

Bleeding can also occur due to a simple hot flash or excessive blood flow, and also people with hemorrhagic leukemia or low blood clotting factors.

- **Treatment**
  Prescription

- **Main point**
  BL-40 (Weizhong 委中)
- He-Sea point of the Bladder channel.
- On the back of the knee, on the midpoint of the transverse crease of the popliteal fossa.

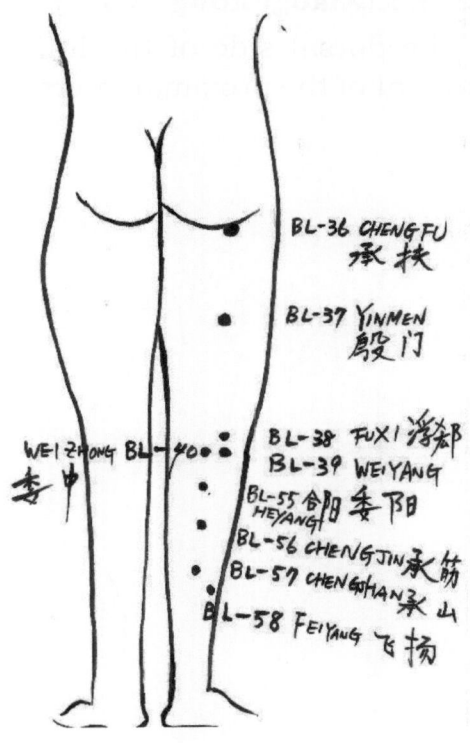

BL-36 CHENGFU 承扶

BL-37 YINMEN 殷门

WEIZHONG BL-40 委中

BL-38 FUXI 浮郄
BL-39 WEIYANG 委阳
BL-55 HEYANG 合阳
BL-56 CHENGJIN 承筋
BL-57 CHENGSHAN 承山
BL-58 FEIYANG 飞扬

5-14 Eye tiredness 眼睛疲劳 Yanjing pilao

It's causing eye strain. Eye fatigue and neck and shoulder fatigue appear together.

- **Treatment**
  Prescription

- **Main point**
  EX-UE6 (Xiaogukong 小骨空)
- On the dorsal side of the little finger, at the midpoint of the proximal interphalangeal joint.

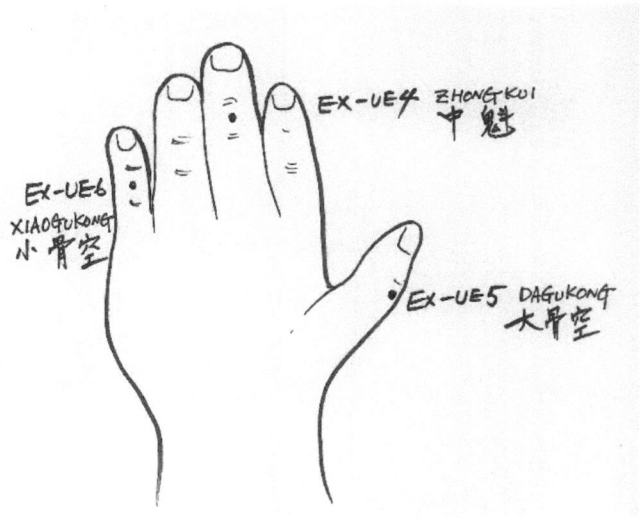

Chapter 6 Miscellaneous

6-1 Obesity 肥胖 Feipang

It refers to excessive accumulation of fat in the body tissues. Clinically, it is divided into Simple and Secondary types.

Simple Obesity: It is due to overeating of greasy, sweet food that exceeds the normal consumption of body heat.

Secondary Obesity: It is caused by hypothalamic pituitary lesions and over-secretion of hydrocortisone.

- **Treatment**
  Prescription

- **Main point**
  REN-4 (Guanyuan 关元)
- Front-Mu point of the Small Intestine.
- On the lower abdomen, 3 cun below the umbilicus.

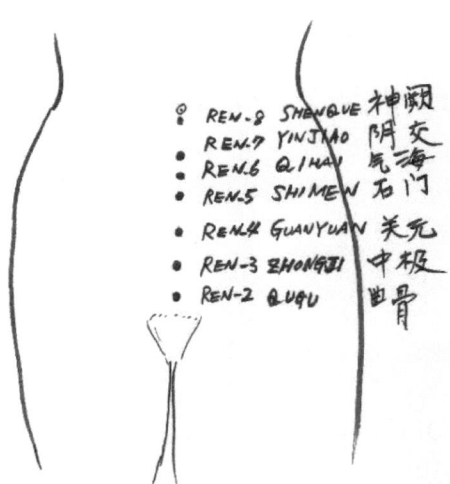

6-2 Sciatica 坐骨神经 Zuogushenjingtong

This is the pain radiating to the sciatic nerve distribution in the hip region, posterior lateral aspect of the leg.

1. Primary Sciatica

   It is characterized by a sudden onset of continuous sharp pain, worsens with cold, alleviates with warmth.

2. Secondary Sciatica

This is a slow onset of pain which may involve primary lesions, radiating pain due to lumbar disc degeneration. The pain is worse with cough, sneezing.

- **Treatment**
  Prescription

- **Main point**
  GB-30 (Huantiao 环跳)
- On the postero-lateral side of the hip joint, one third of the distance between the prominence of the great trochanter and the sacrococcygeal hiatus.

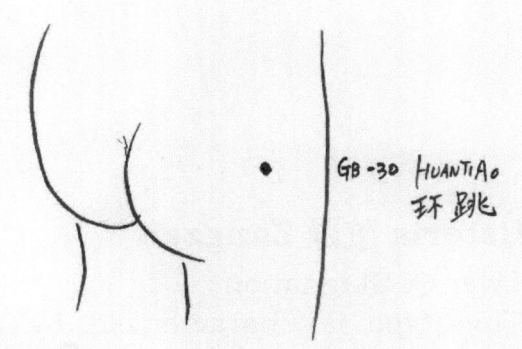

- **Secondary point**
  GB-31 (Fengshi 风市)

- On the lateral midline of the thigh, 7 cun superior to the popliteal crease, when the patient stands erect with the arms hanging down freely, the point is the tip of the middle finger.

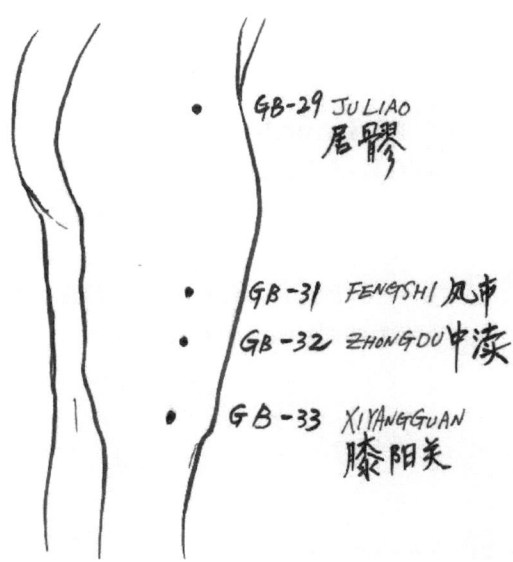

6-3 Histeria 脏躁 Zangzao

1. Liver Qi Stagnation
   This type is characterized by restlessness, mental depression, poor self-control, irritability, red tongue coating, wiry pulse.
2. Emotional Depression

This type is characterized by low spirit, emotional unrest, constant cries with grief or sorrow, pale tongue with white coating, thre. pulse.

- **Treatment**
  Prescription

- **Main point**
  ST-9 (Renying 人迎)
- Level with the tip of Adam apple, on the anterior border of the sternocleidomastoid muscle where the common carotid artery is palpable.

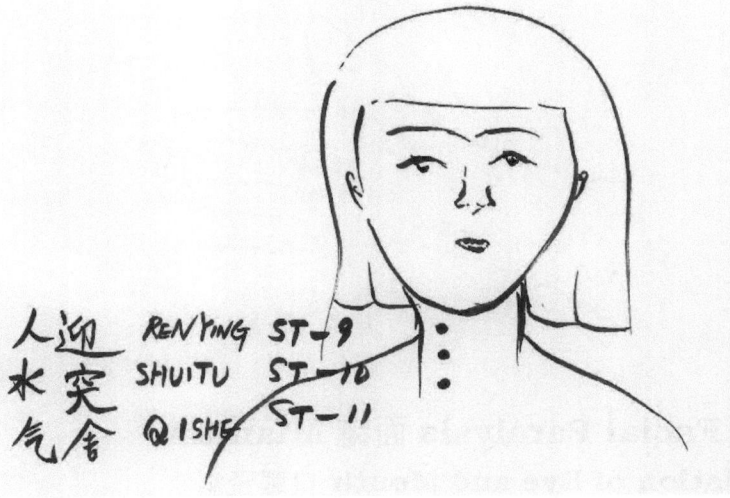

人迎　RENYING　ST-9
水突　SHUITU　ST-10
气舍　QISHE　ST-11

6-4 Facial Spasm 面肌痉挛 Mianjijingluan

This is common in women and refers to spasm on one side of the face. It may be aggravated by fatigue, mental stress, and physical movement.

- **Treatment**
  Prescription
- **Main point**
- **SI-3 (Houxi 后溪)**
- When a loose fist is made, the point on the ulnar side of the hand, at the end of the transverse crease proximal to the fifth metacarpophalangeal joint.

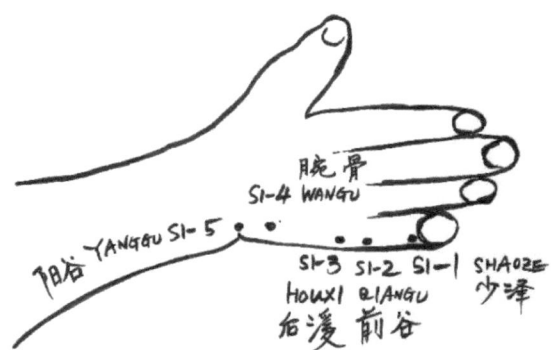

6-5 Facial Paralysis 面瘫 Miantan
Deviation of Eye and Mouth 口眼歪斜 Kouyanwaixie

Deviated mouth and eyes are the common name. The paralysis appears mostly on one side, mostly among young and middle-aged people.

This is caused by weakness of the channels, which are attacked by the exogenous pathogenic wind-cold or wind-heat and led to the flaccidness of muscles by Qi stagnation and blood stasis in the channels of face.

- **Treatment**
  Prescription
- **Main point**
  SJ-17 (Yifeng 翳风)
- Behind the earlobe, in the depression between the mandible and mastoid process.

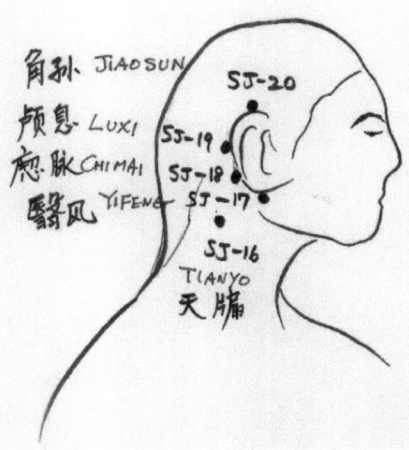

6-6 Hay Fever 花粉过敏 Huafen guomin

Symptoms of hay fever include itchy eyes, watery eyes, runny nose, itchy throat, and sneezing. People with strong immune systems are sensitive to pollen and treat pollen as a foreign substance, causing hay fever.

Additionally, people with other allergies often develop hay fever.

- **Treatment**
  Prescription
- **Main point**
  Li-11 (Quchi 曲池)
- He-Sea point.
- In the depression at the lateral end of the transverse cubital crease.

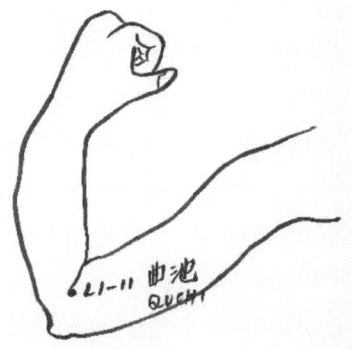

6-7 Hangover, car sickness 宿醉 Su zui、晕车 yunche

Hangover is too much alcohol than liver can handle. The liver processes the alcohol into harmless substances, but too much alcohol, it cannot be processed, and the alcohol remains in the body. Alcohol left in the body also enters the brain. Alcohol that is not broken down by the liver is sent throughout the body through the blood, causing symptoms such as headaches and nausea. It causes various hangover symptoms.

- **Treatment**
  Prescription

- **Main point**
  LIV-1 (Dadun 大敦)
- Jing-Well point.
- On the lateral side of dorsum of the the great toe, 0.1 cun beside the corner of the nail.

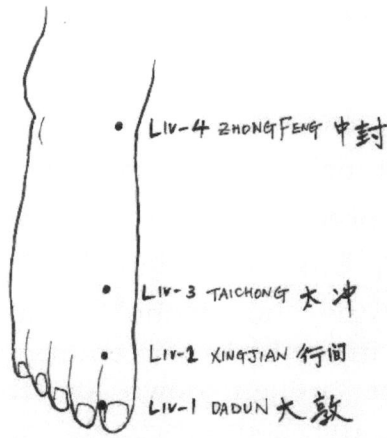

6-8 Heel Pain 脚跟痛 Jiaogen tong

The manifestations are mainly sprain, pain creating on heel contact with the ground and difficult to walk.

- **Treatment**
  Prescription

- **Main point**
  Ashi point

6-9 Regulate excess weight & Metabolic function 调节多余体重和代谢功能.

Tiaojie duoyu tizhong he daixie gongneng

There are two types of fat: body fat and organ fat.Body fat is the subcutaneous fat that accumulates around the stomach, and organ fat is the fat that accumulates in internal organs. Organ fat is the cause of liver and heart diseases. The causes of being overweight are a lack of exercise and too much unbalanced nutrition, as well as overwork and stress.

- **Treatment**
  Prescription
- **Main point**
  SP-8 (Diji 地机)
- Xi-Cleft point of the Spleen channel.
- cun below SP-9 (Yinlingquan 阴陵泉), on the line connecting the tip of the medial malleolus.

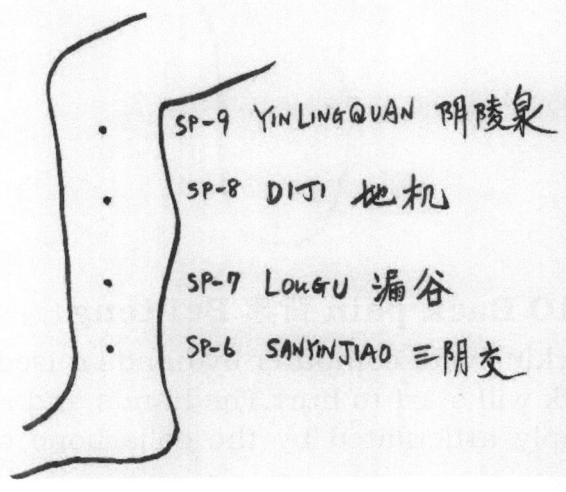

SP-9 YIN LING QUAN 阴陵泉

SP-8 DIJI 地机

SP-7 LOUGU 漏谷

SP-6 SANYINJIAO 三阴交

(1) Lack of Energy and Vitality
- **Main point**
  KI-1 (Yongquan 涌泉)
- Jing-Well point.
- On the sole, at the junction of the anterior one-third and posterior two thirds of the sole, between the second and third metatarsal bones.

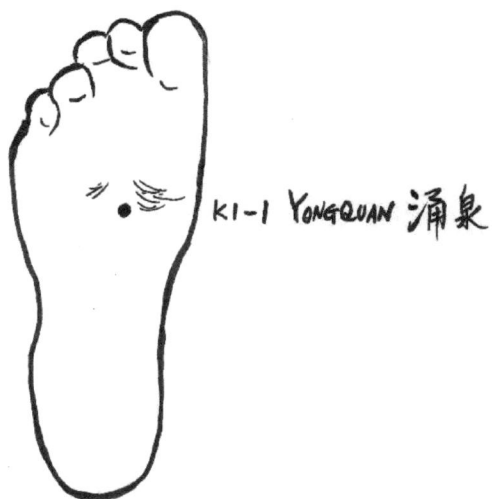

6-10 Back pain 背疼 Bei teng

Working with computer by hands raised in front, the back will start to hurt. The hands and shoulders are simply articulated by the collarbone and shoulder blade, and the muscles and tendons of the neck and shoulders support the weight of the arms, and the psoas muscles also work to balance them. These are overworked muscles, so it's best to give them a break from time to time.

- **Treatment**
  Prescription
- **Main point**
- **P-8 (Laogong 劳宫)**
- On the palm, between the second and third metacarpal bones. When the fist is made, the point is below the tip of the middle finger.
- P-8 improves blood flow to the eyes, neck, and shoulders, eliminating stiffness.

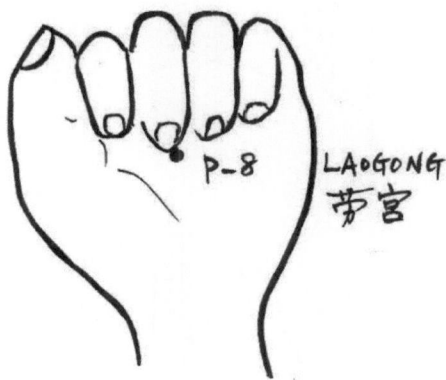

6-11 Occipital Neuralgia 枕部神经痛
Zhen bu shenjing tong

This refers to pain in the occipital and upper cervical areas, and it often caused by infection, neck sprain etc. Its manifestations are pain in the occipital area and upper cervical area, which is induced by awkward movement of the neck, sneezing, and cough.

- **Treatment**
  Prescription
- **Main point**
  GB-20 (Fengchi 风池)
- Below the occiput, at the same level as Du-16 (Fengfu 风府), in the depression between the origins of the sternocleidomastoid and trapezius muscles.

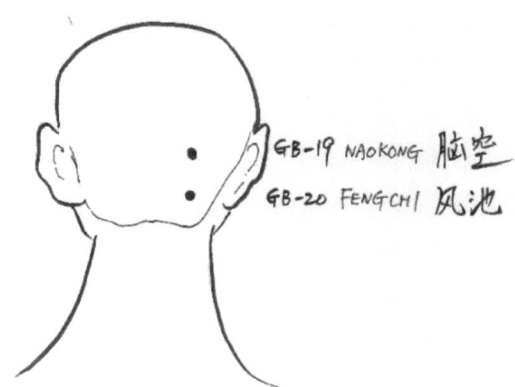

6-12 Pain on Forehead 额头疼痛 Etou tengtong

This is a kind of pain in forehead, supraorbiral bone, migraine, headache syndrome.

- **Treatment**
  Prescription

- **Main point**
  BL-60 (Kunlun 昆仑)
- Behind the ankle joint, in the depression between the prominence of the lateral malleolus.

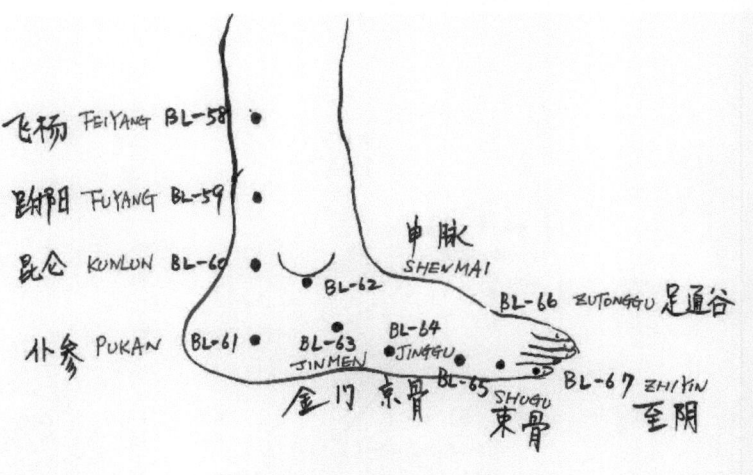

6-13 Trigeminal Neuralgia 三叉神经痛

Sancha shenjing tong

This is characterized by sudden attacks of severe pain in the facial areas, by the trigeminal nerve, maxillary and mandibular divisions. Attacks may recur several times daily.

- **Treatment**
  Prescription

- **Main point**
  SI-19 (Tinggong 听宫)
- In the depression formed when the mouth is open. Anterior to the tragus and posterior to the condyloid process of the mandible.

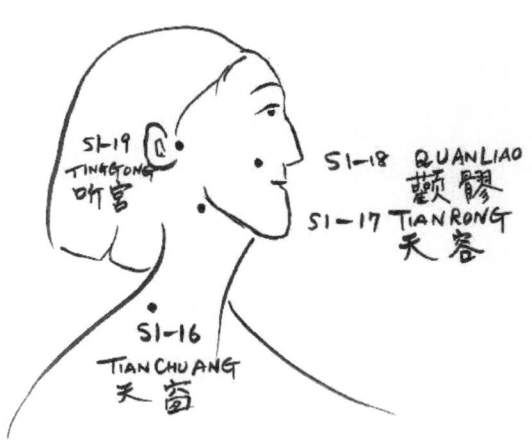

- **Secondary point**
  GB-14 (Yangbai 阳白)
- On the forehead, directly above the pupil, 1 cun superior to the middle of the eyebrow.

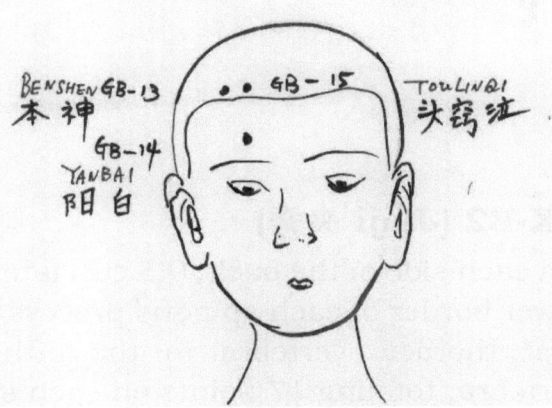

6-14 Cervical Spondylopathy 颈椎病 Jingchuibing

This refers to the cervical vertebra stimulates and oppresses the cervical nerve root, spinal cord, vertebral artery, and sympathetic nerve, causing pain in the around the neck, forearm, shoulder, movement of the head, numbness in the lower limbs, heavy sensation, dizziness, headache.

- **Treatment**

Prescription

- **Main point**

Plum blossom Needle

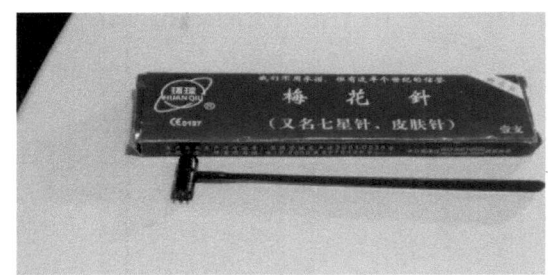

EX-B2 (Jiaji 夹脊)

- On each side of the back, 0.5 cun lateral to the lower border of each spinous process from the first thoracic vertebra to the fifth lumbar vertebra, totaling 17 points on each side.

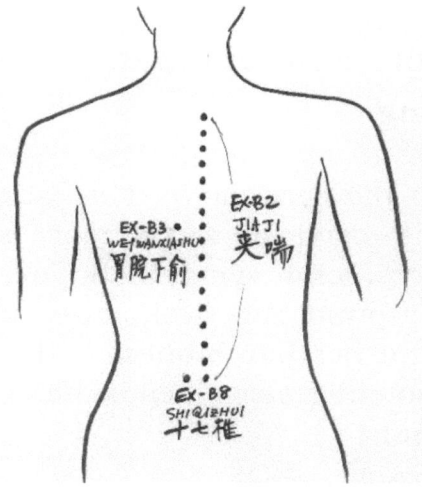

6-15 Knee pain 膝盖疼痛 Xīgai tengtong

Knee pain in young people often comes from injuries such as skiing or traffic accidents. Elderly people may have degenerative knee joints, or they may have a disease in their knees regardless of their age. It may cause lesion to soft tissues such as muscles, tendons, ligaments, etc. Manifestations are painful, tenderness swelling and limitation of movement.

- **Treatment**
  Prescription
- **Main point**
  EX-LE4 (Xiyan 膝眼)
- When the knee is flexed, in the depression medial and lateral side of the patellar ligament, the medial side is called Neixiyan 内膝眼, on the lateral side is called Waixiyan 外膝眼.

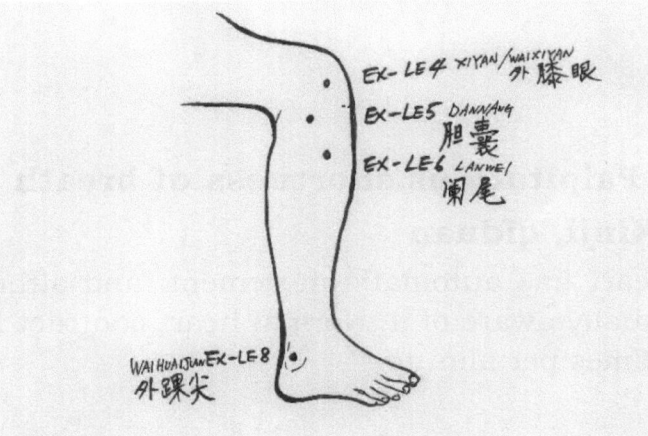

- **Secondary point
  EX-UE5 (Dagukong 大骨空)**
- On the dorsal side of the thumb, at the center of the interphalangeal joint.
- EX-LE4 Xiyan 膝眼 improves blood flow.

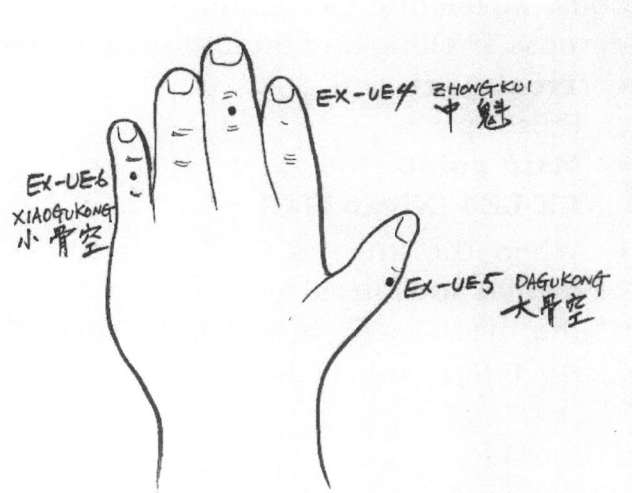

6-16 Palpitations.shortness of breath 心悸、气短 Xinji, qiduan

The heart has automatic movement, and although not usually aware of it. Normal heart contract is 60 to 70 times per minute.

Palpitations are a condition in which you feel your heart beating. Palpitations can occur when the heart rate is increasing, or when the heart rate is normal, but the heartbeat is strong.

It can also occur due to heart disease, anemia, and drinking too much tobacco, coffee, or alcohol.

- **Treatment**
  Prescription
- **Main point**
  P-4 (Ximen 郄门)
- On the palmar side of the forearm, 5 cun above the transverse crease of the wrist, on the line connecting P-3 (Quze 曲泽) and P-7 (Daling 大陵), between the tendons of palmaris longus and flexor carpi radialis.

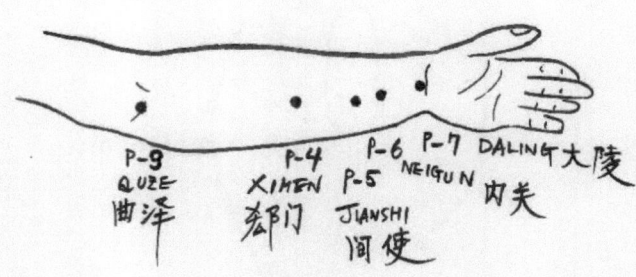

P-9 QUZE 曲泽   P-4 XIMEN 郄门   P-5 JIANSHI 间使   P-6 NEIGUN   P-7 DALING 大陵 内关

6-17 Tiredness 疲倦 Pijuan (overwork)

If patients continue to work with hands raised, patient's back will start to hurt. The hands and shoulders are simply articulated by the clavicle and shoulder blade, and the muscles and tendons of the neck and shoulders support the weight of the arms, and the psoas muscles also work to balance them.

- **Treatment**
  Prescription
- **Main point**
  P-8 (Laogong 劳宫)
- On the palm, between the second and third metacarpal bones. When the fist is made, the point is below the tip of the middle finger.
- P-8 improves blood flow to the eyes, neck, and shoulders, eliminating stiffness.

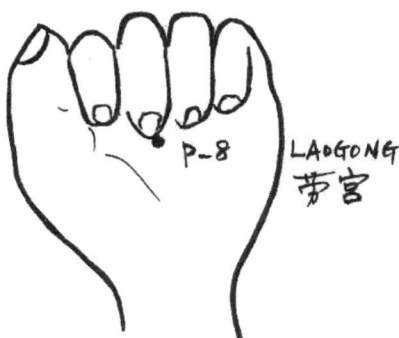

References 参考文献

1. Emi Akimoto, Hand and Foot Acupuncture

2. Chen Decheng, Diseases Treated by Single Point of Acupuncture

3. Sumiko Knudsen, Acupuncture Meridians and Points

4. Sumiko Knudsen, Ear Acupuncture

5. Sumiko Knudsen, Acupuncture for Weight Loss

6. Sumiko Knudsen, Scalp Acupuncture

Other library of Traditional Chinese Medicine by Sumiko Knudsen

1. Acupuncture for Weight Loss
2. Akupunkture til Vægttab
3. Acupuncture Meridians and Points
4. Akupunktur Meridianer og Punkter
5. Ear Acupuncture
6. Øre Akupunktur
7. Body Acupuncture, Clinical Treatment
8. Krop Akupunktur, Klinisk Behandling
9. Acupuncture and Moxibustion
10. Akupunktur og Moxibustion
11. Scalp Acupuncture
12. Hovedbundsakupunktur
13. Hand Acupuncture Clinical Treatment
14. Hånd Akupunktur Klinisk Behandling
15. Foot Acupuncture Clinical Treatment
16. Fod Akupunktur Klinisk Behandling